Capoeira Conditioning

CAPOEIRA CONDITIONING

How to build strength, agility, and cardiovascular fitness using capoeira movements

Gerard Taylor

Photography by Anders Kjaergaard

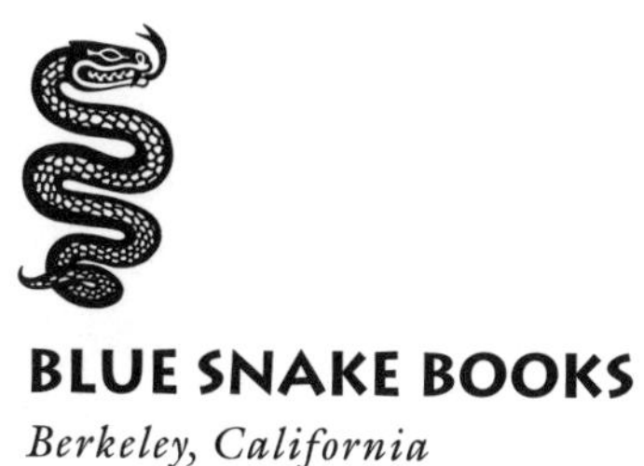

BLUE SNAKE BOOKS

Berkeley, California

Published by Blue Snake Books
Blue Snake Books' publications
are distributed by North Atlantic Books
P.O. Box 12327
Berkeley, California 94712

Cover and text design by Brad Greene
Printed in the United States of America

Capoeira Conditioning is sponsored by the Society for the Study of Native Arts and Sciences, a nonprofit educational corporation whose goals are to develop an educational and cross-cultural perspective linking various scientific, social, and artistic fields; to nurture a holistic view of arts, sciences, humanities, and healing; and to publish and distribute literature on the relationship of mind, body, and nature.

North Atlantic Books' publications are available through most bookstores. For further information, call 800-733-3000 or visit our Web sites at www.northatlanticbooks.com and www.bluesnakebooks.com.

ISBN-13: 978-1-58394-141-6

Library of Congress Cataloging-in-Publication Data

Taylor, Gerard, 1960–
Capoeira conditioning : how to build strength, agility, and cardiovascular fitness using capoeira movements / by Gerard Taylor ; photography by Anders Kjaergaard.
p. cm.
ISBN 1-58394-141-X (pbk.)
1. Capoeira (Dance)—Training. 2. Exercise. I. Title.
GV1796.C145T38 2005
793.3'1981—dc22

2005028921
CIP

5 6 7 8 9 10 11 12 UNITED 14 13 12 11 10 09 08

This book is dedicated to the memory of Derek Taylor, who to my knowledge never did a single workout in his whole life, but sure as hell knew how to write.

Acknowledgments

I'd like to thank Tina, Marit, and Axé, all formados of Oslo Capoeira Klubb, for their patience and hard work while we were putting this book together. Huge thanks to Sue and Anders for commuting between London and Oslo with unusual regularity to take the photos, answer bombardments of e-mails, uncover discrepancies, and amazingly, all remain friends at the end of it.

Acknowledgment to Yvonne Cárdenas of North Atlantic Books for project coordinating, encouragement, and making the copy-editing process a painless experience. "Tusen takk" to Rud Videregående Skole for providing the studio.

Contents

Chapter 3:

The Exercises

Chapter 1

Capoeira Conditioning: What It Is and Why It's Good for You

Strength and Flexibility Capoeira Style

Capoeira is one of the best all-around strength, flexibility, and aerobic exercise systems on the planet. Capoeira gives all the muscle groups of the body a vigorous workout. A person who becomes fit through capoeira movement gains a well-integrated, coordinated musculature, optimal aerobic capacity, and lean, mean cat-like strength and flexibility.

What Is Capoeira Conditioning?

Because it is easy to use words like "fitness," "flexibility," "conditioning," and so on in a very loose way, it is useful to define some of the terms to explain what they mean in the context of capoeira training. First, when we talk about "conditioning" here, it applies to the consistent, all-year-round application of sport-specific physical stress to create a body "conditioned" to the demands of the Brazilian art/sport of capoeira.

Conditioning in sports training is used when trainers refer to exercises done in addition to the actual practice of the sport involved. For example, a football player who trains with weights and sprints is "conditioning" his body for playing football. It is a rare athlete today who trains for their sport solely by doing the sport itself, and most sports training involves some level of conditioning training.

Conditioning for Capoeira "Fitness"

"Fitness" is commonly used in the popular media and modern language to describe a general state of well-being and health. In sports it is often more narrowly defined. In this context fitness relates specifically to a sport and a set of physical abilities or skills. A sub-2.15 marathon runner is not "fit" to deadlift 600 pounds of iron, and a world-class power lifter is not "fit" to run a sub-28-minute 10,000 meters. Using our narrow definition, neither athlete would be "fit" to perform any number of movements on the gymnastics balance beam. The Olympic gymnast would not be "fit" for sumo wrestling, and so forth.

When we talk of "total" fitness, this must encompass a set of necessary components so that the term "total" is not meaningless hyperbole. The range of skills and functions that would have to be included for total fitness are:

Strength. Strength is a muscle's ability to contract against the resistance of an external object (a weight) or one's own body weight.

Power. Slightly different from strength, power relates to the absolute muscular contraction achieved in a dynamic explosion of movement such as a high jump, a kick, or a lift. Power utilizes strength within an explosive burst of energy.

Agility. Agility is often confused with flexibility although it's a different thing. Agility encompasses the possibility of executing power movements in rapidly changing directions. Imagine an acrobat performing forward and back saltos in quick combination, a football player sprinting between opposing players, or a capoeirista weaving in and out of the other's game to the rhythm of music.

Balance. The close cousin of agility, balance involves one's muscular control of the body position, either statically (as in a handstand) or kinesthetically (for example, control and balance of the position of voluntary muscles and the whole body during an acrobatic movement).

Flexibility. The Oxford Dictionary definition of flexible is: "able to bend without breaking; pliable; pliant." The dictionary also defines "flexile" as "supple or mobile." In terms of our total fitness paradigm, there are different types of flexibility.

Dynamic flexibility, also known as kinetic flexibility, encompasses an ability to perform dynamic (kinetic) muscular movements of a limb through the fullest range of motion possible in relation to the joints. Static-active flexibility allows for first assuming and then maintaining extended positions of a limb while using only the muscles of one's body and no external apparatus. Static-passive flexibility allows one to assume positions of the limbs (for instance, side splits) and hold them using body weight, the limbs, and an external apparatus (in the case of side splits, the floor).

If you hold your leg up to your ear, without using your hands, that is static-active flexibility; if you hold it in this position with your hand, this is static-passive flexibility; and if you kick the leg up through a similar range of motion, this is dynamic or kinetic flexibility.

Cardiovascular Endurance. This is the heart's ability to circulate blood to muscles during strenuous physical activity, and the muscles' fitness to use the blood circulated via the blood vessels. "Cardio" means heart, and "vascular" means blood vessels. The vascular system includes arteries, veins, and capillaries, which will be discussed later.

Coordination. This is the state of integration of all the other components into a single functional package so that grace, economy of movement, and physical efficiency are achieved at a high level.

Total Fitness

This is a sport-specific conditioning program for capoeira suitable for capoeira players and non-capoeira players alike.

The reason why a sport-specific conditioning program for capoeira is so very effective is because the game of capoeira develops all **"the big 7"** of a total fitness regime: strength, power, agility, balance, flexibility, cardiovascular endurance, and coordination. This is why I felt justified writing, "Capoeira is one of the best all-around strength, flexibility, and aerobic exercise systems on the planet." Because it is, from whichever angle one looks at it.

Jogo: Game

Roda: Circle where capoeira is played

Rep: Repetitions of a particular exercise

Set: A group of repetitions of a particular exercise

Who Is Capoeira Conditioning For?

The short answer is everybody. Capoeira is for women and men, boys and girls, young and old, fit and presently thinking of becoming fit. This book is designed to provide exercises that are based purely on the movements of capoeira. This means that the body is "conditioned" for actually playing the game of capoeira and is also conditioned for the game of life for those who are not capoeira players.

Capoeira conditioning will work effectively for people who have never done capoeira but would like to use these capoeira training movements to get in the best shape of their lives.

"Really?" you may be asking. "The best shape of my life?"

By doing these simple capoeira conditioning exercises, you can develop and maintain a high level of useable fitness for everyday living. If you are looking for a capoeira club and intend to get in shape prior to starting, this book is also for you.

Athletes and fitness enthusiasts in a wide range of sports will find these exercises highly beneficial for loosening up the tightness sometimes caused by sports training. The rhythmic and physical components of capoeira conditioning are perfect for cross-training. Mané Garrincha, Pelé's legendary contemporary on the Brazilian national soccer team, had amazing "jogo de cintura" (agility of his waist) and dribbling skills often said to derive from his practice of capoeira.

These exercises are a very useful tool for people who already do capoeira and would like to stay in great condition when traveling or otherwise not able to attend regular classes for one reason or another. Anyone who does capoeira will know how dispiriting it can be entering the roda after time away, because the body feels heavy, the feet are slow, and coordination has decreased. To maintain year-round fitness for the game even during enforced time off, these exercises provide a solution. Many can also be applied to stay in shape while recuperating from injury, so a player can choose specific exercises to train while giving an injured body area a rest.

Capoeira conditioning is a capoeira "fitness pill" to take daily to ensure the machine (that is, your body) is ready to play the game of capoeira or life anytime, anyplace, 365 days a year.

It should be stressed that you can't learn capoeira from a book. That is a basic truth.

To learn the holistic art form, music, strategies, and philosophy, an individual will need a qualified teacher and fellow students to play the game with. Yet if you follow these guidelines you can use this book to transform yourself into someone with the "panther-like" fitness and physical condition of a capoeira player, ***even if you don't know how to do capoeira.***

Please note that even though all the exercises in capoeira conditioning are safe and tried and tested, it is a sensible idea before embarking on any exercise program to consult your physician and discuss what you're going to do. This is particularly true if you have received treatment for problems with your vertebrae or are presently working with an osteopath or chiropractor for any spinal or neck injuries.

How Much Time Will You Need to Spend on These Exercises?

People often overestimate the length of time that is needed to get into great condition. This is in some ways the legacy of the marathon running revolution of the past quarter century, which basically involved running long distances incredibly slowly. It is not the intention here to knock running, which is an excellent exercise, fun, (and totally free). It is not, unfortunately, a particularly well-balanced exercise. Yes, our ancestors ran long distances, though not on concrete and tarmac.

The jogging or marathon boom, even the mass-participation fun-run and 10k mini-boom, often meant at least half an hour of running every day, with a regular one- to two-hour "Long Steady Distance" (LSD) run on Sunday morning. Speak to any runner long enough and you'll be treated to a compendium of past injuries that reads like a logbook from the accident and emergency ward.

Currently, a lot of people are extremely busy and want to build

overall fitness without having to use vast amounts of time or running great distances. Capoeira conditioning is a more well-rounded solution.

It can also effectively replace a run on a rest day and provide a brilliant cross-training session to utilize the muscles in a completely new and refreshing way to help avoid the repetitive stress injuries often associated with running.

The running boom was closely followed by a weight-training boom, which has also resulted in people spending large amounts of time in the gym effectively doing nothing but looking in the mirror while they wait for their muscles to recover between sets. Most fitness enthusiasts have been there—pushing the iron, waiting distractedly for those stubborn varmints to grow, and standing patiently in line hoping to get a shot at the peck deck sometime before the end of the next century. Any exercise system that involves spending more time standing in line feeling impatient than training needs a rethink and some fine-tuning.

Train Smart, Not Long.

Did you know that Roger Bannister cracked the 4-minute mile on half-hour training sessions three or four times a week? He did this to fit his world record training in with his university studies. Even when he decided to increase his workload for the final push in breaking through one of athletics' greatest barriers, he jogged 10 minutes to the local track, knocked off ten 400-meter sprint intervals of around 60 seconds each, with two minutes' rest in between. A 10-minute jog back to the hospital saw the whole session finished in 48 minutes, leaving him 12 minutes to eat his lunch out of an hour's lunch break. Did you know that Dr. Franco Columbo won a Mr. Olympia title on just a fraction of the gym time used by his competitors so that it wouldn't disrupt his chiropractic studies? These were competitors who trained smart rather than long and this is the way many people would rather train in today's world.

Most people spend time juggling various different activities, multitasking, often commuting, attempting to devote quality time to family, and so forth. Have you ever tried to justify that two-hour run or trip to the gym to a stressed-out partner who really doesn't understand exactly why a six-pack takes precedence over family life or an occasional meal together? And yet you've been behind the desk all day and if you don't sweat out some of that energy soon you know you're going to explode!

Capoeira conditioning can be fitted easily into a corner of the day and will have you glistening with sweat and pumping oxygen-infused blood in 15 minutes flat. No one even needs to know it ever happened. You'll be ready for a shower and can relax and get on with your life confident that training-wise, today was mission accomplished. That's a promise.

You'll experience a whole body workout and there is no down-time. You can do a very effective conditioning session in as little as 15 minutes of active training. To many people this sounds unrealistic, and yet it's completely logical! All you need is a shift in consciousness as to whether all that LSD or "mirror-time" is really necessary.

The Fat-Burning Power of High-Intensity Interval Training

In a three-week study conducted at McMaster University in Canada by Professor Martin Gibala, twenty-three individuals were thoroughly tested for different fitness regimes. One group cycled for two hours at a moderate, easy pace. The second group did 10 minutes of cycling per training session, including a few 60-second bursts.

The third group went flat out for just four 30-second periods, interspersed with a 4-minute rest between each burst.

So the differentiated training was of a two-hour duration for one group, a 10-minute duration for another, and a 2-minute active duration for the third.

At the beginning, each participant did an 18.6-mile cycle time trial, and they concluded with the same at the end, to measure and compare progress after three weeks. The results were all exactly the same. Despite the huge training time difference, everyone had improved to the same degree. Further, their VO2 Max (the rate at which their muscles absorbed oxygen) had also improved by an identical amount. Gibala concluded: "Short bouts of very intense exercise improved muscle health and performance comparable to several weeks of endurance training."

The type of training Dr. Gibala was testing is called "high-intensity interval training" (HIIT). Today, more and more fitness-minded people are realizing that short, intense exercise sessions are the way to go for the best return on a training investment. An important paper, by Angelo Tremblay and Claude Bouchard, was published in 1995 and came to similar conclusions as those of Professor Gibala. Over a six-week period, a "sprint" cycle group dropped over three times as much body fat as a slow, aerobic group. This was despite burning only approximately half the calories during the active exercise. The aerobic group did 45-minute workouts five times a week at a steady medium pace. The high-intensity interval training group did only 30 minutes (including warm-up and cool-off recovery) three times per week. Yet they burned off triple the body fat!

Why is it that HIIT works so effectively? It is because of a state known as "excessive post-exercise oxygen consumption." In practice, you have a much higher post-exercise metabolic rate following the intervals. In 1996, a University of Alabama study found a higher rate of metabolism (meaning calorie and fat burning) even 24 hours after a high-intensity interval training session. People who want to retain muscle bulk but lose fat love HIIT because it has the effect of increasing calorie consumption dramatically without using muscle as actual fuel.

There is one proviso here. It is a fact that HIIT works far more effectively for people already in good shape. Aerobic training is great for building initial stamina and endurance. So the rule of thumb is: take it easy. Build up your fitness with regular 15- to 30-minute sessions and then experiment with some all-out mega-energy bursts of 30 seconds' duration every few minutes (for example, four flat-out 30-second bursts embedded within a 15-minute training session). This will kick-start the excess post-exercise oxygen consumption (EPOC) effect.

Note: When we talk of a mega-energy burst, we are in reality saying work flat-out, peak intensity for 30 seconds. Half a minute may seem like child's play, but once you've experienced 30 seconds of no-holds-barred exercise bedlam, you'll never knock it again.

You can reproduce this with many of the exercises in the capoeira conditioning system as long as you have the guts to push yourself to the limit for those short but peak-experience 30 seconds of life.

Try it now. Put your hand on your heart and feel it. Set your stopwatch, hit the floor, and cobra-run sprint (see exercise No. 40) at top speed for 30 seconds. Feel your heart again. In the capoeira conditioning system when you are resting you are still conditioning your body with capoeira movements, so as you recover now, try some gentle bridging or side bends while you wait for your heart to stop trying to bomb its way out of your rib cage.

What Makes Capoeira Conditioning So Effective?

Our bodies are like elastic putty that is shaped by everything we do throughout our lives. For many of us, even during our teenage years, this putty begins to harden and become less pliable. Our range of movement decreases while our aches and pains increase week by week. We get tired more easily and we're afflicted by all kinds of small nagging mental or physical discomforts. We put it down to aging.

Twenty-four hours a day, seven days a week, the force of gravity drags on our musculature, skeleton, and internal organs. Any imbalances are reinforced by gravity. Our inner universe (that is, all that stuff we don't see just under our skin)—muscles, organs, bones, blood vessels, and nerves—is covered with and connected by a thin fiber of connective tissue called "fascia." Imagine it as an elasticized matrix (sometimes described as a cobweb) stretched like a sheath over everything else. Over the years, from the moment of birth, our movements affect the shape of this fascia.

It is made up largely of a protein called "collagen." Collagen can be beautifully soft like jelly, or hard and unyielding like rawhide. As we travel through life, picking up injuries, developing incorrect postural habits, our fascia is constantly adapting, in some parts hardening and compensating in ways that tighten us up. If gravity, injuries, misuse, unnatural posture, and misaligned joints have thrown our body out of balance, the hardening fascia will hold the whole structure together with the same imbalances left unchecked.

Repetitive training may reinforce imbalances within the body. A 10-mile run with the head thrust forward, landing more heavily on one ankle than the other, with a rib cage not fully involved in the process of breathing, might promote bodily stress rather than optimal health. Similar problems can occur when repetitively lifting weights with an imbalanced posture.

The fascia is educated by the way we use our bodies. An oft-used example is crossing our arms. Please try it now. See what you do?

The arms are automatically crossed in exactly the same way you have always crossed them. You've probably done it like that for years. Try doing it with the other arm on top and it feels weird. That's the fascia in action, like a body memory. It is the same for many of the movements we all perform throughout the day, from standing, to walking, eating, brushing our teeth, even to making love. If we want to free up our frame, we can begin by remolding the fascia.

Now the Good News

The beauty of capoeira conditioning is its potential for restoring the body to balance. This means that as an exercise system it is complete within itself and needs no supplementary elements. This is why it's the real McCoy as a cross-training system and for whole-body workouts with no need for equipment, special clothes, shoes, machinery, gym membership, pills, potions, or performance-enhancing drugs.

Capoeira exercises provide an effective counter to movement patterns and possibly bad habits we may have been practicing since we were in diapers. The range of movement is so varied that the fascia is stretched out, elongated, pulled, and loosened from every conceivable angle. Before returning to the fascia, an overview about how the musculature, skeletal structure, and breathing tie in will be useful here.

About Breathing

You'll notice that during many of the exercises in this book, deep nasal breathing is recommended. Breathing is one of the most important elements of any effective fitness program, and the aim of deep nasal "diaphragmatic" breathing is to draw air into the lower lobes of the lungs first for a more effective oxygen exchange while exercising.

The Diaphragm

This is a flat muscle at the base of the lungs. Like all muscles, the diaphragm will be strengthened with correct training. When we inhale, the diaphragm contracts and the lower rib cage expands, as does the abdomen. When we exhale, the lungs recoil, somewhat like an inflated balloon whose air is escaping.

If we breathe only through our mouths in shallow breaths, we fill the middle and upper part of our lungs with oxygen, but hardly ever reach the lower lobes, where the best blood supply is. The human, like most mammals, is made for nasal breathing. Babies breathe through their noses and only turn to mouth breathing when the nose gets too congested to provide sufficient oxygen. We learn mouth breathing as we grow up and by the time we are adults, the majority of people in our society are shallow breathers. If we inhale shallow breaths, paradoxically we tend to take in too much oxygen, and never achieve a correct balance between the oxygen and carbon dioxide (CO_2) in our lungs.

At first you may well find it more difficult to get the air you need during exercise when breathing through your nose. This is a matter of practice. If you are already in good shape, when you start capoeira conditioning you may need to work at a slightly reduced intensity when breathing only through the nose. After practicing the method for some time, you'll be able to train at a high intensity level, as you engage the lowest lobes of your lungs and take stress off your heart. You can experiment. If you really want to go "eyeballs out" you might try inhaling through the nose and exhaling through the mouth. Purists can use the nose for the whole enchilada (the full respiration of inhalation and exhalation).

During strenuous exercise, when you gulp in masses of oxygen through your mouth, it goes to the upper and middle part of your lungs. Your heart beats rapidly to push the blood through your lungs more quickly to feed your muscles, but this gives the blood less time in the lungs, and virtually no time in the lower lobes of your lungs for really effective oxygen exchange. Deep, diaphragmatic nasal breathing will deliver oxygen to your lungs more slowly, but more effectively, because it will deliver it to the blood-rich lower lobes, for a more effective oxygen exchange.

The emphasis in capoeira conditioning is to use the abdominal muscles to expel air from your lungs as you exhale. After you have contracted your abs and exhaled forcefully, the inhalation is automatic.

Nasal Breathing Exercise

Try this lying on your back just to get the feel of it. Keep your mouth closed all the way through the exercise. Lie down on your back and suck in a long, steady inhalation of air through your nose. When you have taken in as much air as you can, hold your breath for a few seconds. Then exhale through your nose in an even longer steady breath, tightening your abdominal muscles at the end of the breath to expel air from your lungs effectively, as if you're trying to squeeze your navel back toward your spine. When you can exhale no more air, relax completely and see how your inhalation occurs automatically as your body sucks the air in through your nose without your having to consciously control it.

A shallow breather will respirate twelve or more times in a minute, but a deep breather can easily reduce this amount to four or even two times per minute.

Breathing Is a Workout

When we habitually breathe deeply through the natural apparatus for respiration (the nose), it is an incredibly effective workout for our abdominal muscles, our lungs, diaphragm, spine, and rib cage. The rib cage should expand and then contract with each breath. Our rib cage actually widens as we inhale, and our body lengthens. When we exhale, it contracts, softens, and relaxes. If we don't breathe deeply, the ribs don't move dynamically, and the whole trunk gradually stiffens up and loses flexibility.

Think of your torso as a round, upright tube with three horizontal sections. At the base is the pelvic floor, the ceiling is the dome of your upper rib cage, and the middle is the diaphragm muscle. Beneath the diaphragm is the abdominal cavity and many important organs, including your kidneys. Fitting snugly above the diaphragm is the thorax (chest cavity), in which the heart and lungs are contained.

Our ribs are attached to the spine; with correct deep breathing the ribs gently massage the spine and internal organs. When we breathe deeply during many of the capoeira movements shown in this book, this massage effect is heightened. If an exercise is a static pose, remember always that we are never literally static. Breath is movement, and every deep respiration increases the flexibility of your rib cage and spine, which will obviously increase your overall mobility and fitness for capoeira and many other activities.

Two-Way Benefits

During strenuous capoeira movement, inside the body there is a parallel game going on, in which accessory muscles from the legs to the jaw are working toward opening and closing the chest cavity for greater respiration. Everything is geared toward expanding the chest. If we view the body as a mechanical system, this task is made easier when the rib cage, spine, hips, and shoulders are loose and flexible.

Right there in the middle of your chest is the heart. Think of it as a pump, and in a long and even otherwise uneventful lifetime it will beat an average of two and a half billion times without ever stopping to take a rest. The heart pumps out around 10 pints of blood a minute when you're resting and more than 70 pints per minute during strenuous exercise.

The heart is a muscle about the size of a closed fist. It sits right there atop the diaphragm and between the lungs; it isn't just a blob of pumping mass doing its thing independently from the rest of our structure. The heart moves and changes shape with every single one of the millions of breaths we take. Bad posture and structural imbalances may compress the heart and will also affect the diaphragm on which it is supported. On the other hand, good posture and a fully expanding and contracting rib cage and spine will encourage optimal heart function.

During our respiration cycle various systems are working simultaneously to facilitate blood circulation. First there is the coronary system, which involves the movement of blood between the four main cavities of the heart (the atria and ventricles). Then there is the pulmonary system, which is responsible for the circulation of blood between the heart and the lungs. Last is the systematic circulation, which involves the transport of blood to all the other organs of the body besides the heart and lungs.

Blood circulation throughout the body happens via blood vessels (veins, arteries, and capillaries). There are around 100,000 miles of blood vessels in an average adult body! These lie across or underneath, or are surrounded by muscles. Relaxed muscles that are not stiff and overcontracted won't squeeze and pinch the blood vessels, meaning they transport blood more effectively.

Via blood vessels (veins), waste-infused blood enters the heart. By the action of the coronary system the heart pumps blood into the pulmonary artery. This leads to the lungs. The waste-infused blood contains carbon dioxide and other gases. Within the lungs, the miraculous switch occurs.

Imagine you've just taken a deep breath of oxygen. This air passes through various tubes—first the larynx and then the trachea, a tube that enters the chest cavity. The trachea branches off into two thinner tubes (the bronchi), which in turn subdivide into bronchioles that lead into the lungs. The oxygen you have inhaled passes through the bronchial tubes and into even thinner tubes, which connect to minuscule sacs (alveoli), of which there are approximately 600 million in an average pair of lungs. Once in the alveoli, the oxygen floods through capillaries into arterial blood (which is there in more abundance in the lowest lobes of your lungs).

The CO_2 infused blood by now has also been released into the alveoli, and as you exhale that CO_2 leaves your lungs via exactly the same route the oxygen entered. The oxygen-rich blood from your lungs will now enter the heart again via the pulmonary system, and from there once more do its rounds of your body via the blood vessels. And so it goes on, from the moment of your birth, to the last breath you ever take.

Use this miracle within your chest well and it will serve you all the days of your life. Cramp yourself up with bad posture, eat high-fat food, and never exercise, or even send tar, nicotine, and carbon monoxide flowing into your lungs along with the oxygen, and things may not be so sweet.

Full-Body Breathing

One last pointer concerning breathing. In our exercise, we took an abdominal tension breath, which is a good start for practicing nasal breathing. As you do capoeira conditioning, try to develop your body awareness to a new level.

Remember at the beginning of this section we talked about the "fascia," that thin network of connective tissue enveloping the bones, muscles, and joints, holding everything together. Because it is a colloid, the collagen in the fascia can turn from liquid to solid and from solid to liquid. Tensions within our bodies, which may become chronic, will also have the tendency to shorten and harden the fascia.

Obviously it is not necessary to be imagining the internal universe of your body all the time while exercising, though from time to time as you perform these exercises, get really quiet and aware of your breathing. Be aware of your diaphragm rising and flattening as you exhale and inhale. Be aware that the fascia matrix responds to the action of your muscles as you breathe. Be conscious that this occurs all over your body, from the top of your head to the soles of your feet. So breathe long and deep while your ribs rise and fall, expand and contract, your spine lengthening and releasing naturally by the action of your breathing. Remain relaxed, even when you are doing exercises that may seem at first to be primarily strength building; consider all the movements to really be a stretch.

Chapter 2

The Training

Core Movements

There will be some emphasis in the training on what may be termed "core movements" in capoeira conditioning. "Core movements" in this context means that they are the essential building blocks of this training system. Another way the word "core" is used in relation to training is when we talk about the body's "core," which usually refers to the abdominal muscles and the muscles of the lower back. Coincidentally, some of the core movements will condition the body's "core" very effectively, but that isn't why they are called core movements.

The core movements represent basic, simple exercises that will work the muscles and joints you would mainly be using during the game of capoeira. As core movements, if you did absolutely nothing else, these movements alone, done in sufficient quantity, will keep you in great shape both for playing the game of capoeira and for living life.

The core movements are:

(No. 3) Cocorinha (squats)

(No. 14) Ponte (back bridge)

(No. 25) Aú Normal (cartwheel)

(No. 33/34) Plantanda Bananeira (handstand) and Bananeira Push-Up

Later on you will find a Training Effects Chart to guide you to particular exercises that emphasize different areas of overall conditioning. Exercises that relate to core movements will be shown in bold print and in parentheses. If numbers other than (3), (14), (25), and (33/34) are shown in bold print, it is because they are exercises closely related to the core movements. For example, although No. 14, the Ponte (back bridge), is the core movement, No. 15 (a Ponte back bridge with the heels raised) and No. 18 (Ponte back bridge push-ups) will also be shown in bold print, as they are such close relatives and may be useful for those who find bridges with heels down difficult, or who want to up the ante with some moving bridges.

Cocorinha Squats

The squat increases energy flow, and helps free up tensions in the pelvis and perineal floor. It gives a gentle stretch to the body's major muscles. The squat is highly regarded in bodywork systems such as "polarity theory." It is used to ground us to the earth and indeed forms the basis of the "polarity" exercise forms. The "utkatasana" or "hunkering posture" is recorded as one of the 32 asanas that are the most important in hatha yoga. The way it is sometimes done, with raised heels and the knees a little apart, is perfect for people whose ankles are too tight to handle the full cocorinha with heels pressed into the floor.

The cocorinha squat can also be utilized to give us an incredible leg and cardio workout. Many combat/sport systems base exercise sessions on the squat. Ken Shamrock is known to use high-repetition squats of up to 500 to get his fighters in shape in his training headquarters, "The Lion's Den." "The Hindu Squat," a special and highly effective variation, has been popularized by the catch wrestling and kung fu world champion Matt Furey.

In arts where amazing leg strength, suppleness, and springiness for jumping are needed, such as ballet, high repetitions of the half knee bend (demi plié) and full knee bend (grand plié) are vital for building dynamic power in the thighs and buttocks, and for strengthening the Achilles tendon and ankle too. Many worldwide folk dances and styles that require extreme athleticism and agility also emphasize thigh power derived from squats. To name but two: Russian Cossack dancing and the Norwegian Halling dance, which feature leaps, very high kicks, and somersaults, include many variations of the squatting position as their integral characteristic. "Plyometrics," the training system that is used where jump height is increased for sports like basketball or the high jump, also emphasizes the type of leg conditioning that can be built from squats, jump squats, bunny hops, and exercises of that type.

In other words, if you want great capoeira conditioning, make friends with the cocorinha.

Ponte: The Back Bridge

The back bridge in capoeira conditioning prepares the body for many movements within the game (such as moenda, macaco, gato, and walkovers). For those who don't do capoeira itself, the back bridge may be familiar if you have tried judo, gymnastics, yoga, or wrestling. In India it's called chakrasana ("wheel posture") and is said to be one of the most therapeutic postures in yoga. One of Mestre Bimba's entrance tests at his Capoeira Academy was the prospective student's fitness to perform a back bridge.

It will enlarge your rib cage and increase thoracic mobility. It helps trim away fat from your abs and thighs, and is beneficial for the nervous system, glands, and reproductive organs. It will also build strength in your ankles and wrists and because of the strong arch to your spine it will stretch out the whole front of your body and strengthen the hips. There are variations of this movement in capoeira conditioning, though it is the static arms extended back bridge that is the core movement to concentrate on.

Aú Normal (Cartwheel)

The basic cartwheel is one of the first "acrobatic" movements many people in capoeira learn. It is a natural movement of the human body, as is witnessed by its popularity among young children, who throw themselves about with it almost as soon as they have learned to walk. It is a playful movement and seemingly simple; however, the aú is also very subtle and versatile. By turning this inverted wheel you can build coordination and balance skills, build stamina, trim your waist, strengthen the arms and shoulders, and it forms the basis of many other types of aú in the game of capoeira—from aú batendo, to aú coice, aú quebrada, aú espinha, and many others. Aú batendo is a cartwheel with a downward "martelo"—hammer kick—in the middle of the movement. Aú coice is a cartwheel that delivers a two-footed "mule kick." Aú quebrada means an aú with a smash, wherein one straight leg is kicked forward and inward toward the capoeirista's body, while they are inverted on one hand. This is sometimes called "bico de papagaio" too. The aú espinha is an aú wherein the spine and hips are rotated during the movement so that the hips are centered and facing upward and forward.

Plantanda Bananeira (Handstand) and Bananeira Push-Up

These are more of those universal movements that break down barriers between different disciplines. The handstand forms the basis of any number of gymnastic and acrobatic movements and is an essential component of the game of capoeira. Players who can't hold a full, static handstand will nonetheless often do movements that utilize, however fleetingly, the position of the bananeira. The handstand is a key component of gymnastic training, and the handstand push-up is one of the best exercises for total torso and shoulder strength. Gymnast and author Dan Millman described in *Way of the Peaceful Warrior* how he built his strength back up again after breaking his leg in a serious motorcycle crash: **"I began a program of exercise, slowly at first, then more intensely. . . . I carefully pressed up to handstands, then pumped up and down, again and again, puffing with exertion until every muscle had worked to its limit and my body glistened. . . ."*** He went on to become a National Collegiate Gymnastic champion and World Trampoline champion.

Once again, the movement is used in yoga, and is known as the "balancing tree posture." Bananeira comes with good credentials, and if you want to get strong with a capital S without laying hands on a barbell, this is the movement for you.

Workout Menu

The following combination ideas are just a guideline. Once you have some practice with capoeira conditioning, or if you are already a capoeirista, you can put together your own combinations of exercises to suit your schedule and the time you wish to devote to capoeira conditioning from day to day. Given here are some sequences of exercises that provide an all-around workout, and some sequences that you may enjoy if you want to put special emphasis on one particular aspect of fitness—for example, "arm, back, and shoulder capoeira conditioning," "capoeira leg conditioning," and so on.

---

* Millman, Dan. *Way of the Peaceful Warrior: A Book That Changes Lives* (Tiburon, Calif.: H. J. Kramer/New World Library, 2000), p. 97.

7½-Minute Capoeira Conditioning Maintenance Workouts

When you are strapped for time, you can do one of these at any time of day, or combine them for 15-minute workouts, or do one in the morning and one in the evening—whatever suits your schedule.

Leg and aerobic workout

No. 3 Cocorinha Squats

Do 250 cocorinha squats in 7½ minutes. If you have hardly any time to spare, but you still want to do something, this will give you an effective session in minimum time.

Leg, back, and shoulder workout

No. 3 Cocorinha Squats

No. 8 Wrist Rotation

No. 34 Bananeira Push-Ups

For a full body blaster, do five rapid sets of 50 cocorinha squats (while rotating your wrists to warm them up) alternating with five sets of bananeira push-ups. If you work quickly and methodically, this should be possible to achieve in 10 minutes.

Legs, back, shoulders, hips, and high-intensity cardiovascular workout

No. 40 Cobra Running

No. 20 No Cheat Bridge

Do 30 seconds of cobra running explosively and at a flat-out pace. Alternate with two rounds of no cheat bridge, back and forth. Repeat the cycle of movements, switching from 30 seconds of cobra running flat out to no cheat bridge for four complete turns. This workout can be completed in 7½ to 10 minutes total.

Arms, shoulders, waist, and aerobic workout

No. 25 Aú Normal

Do as many of this movement as you can in 7½ minutes. Move rhythmically from side to side without stopping. If you need to take a break, simply do a few No. 4 ginga, then continue.

Legs, arms, shoulders, and waist workout

No. 25 Aú Normal + No. 3 Cocorinha Squats

Au normal to the right. Drop into a cocorinha squat, then up into an aú normal to the left, then cocorinha and to the right again. Move back and forth rhythmically for 7½ minutes and you'll be breathing hard, so take it easy. This will tone up your muscles, give you an aerobic workout, and add to your springiness within the roda.

Legs, back, and shoulder workout

No. 8 Wrist Rotation

No. 3 Cocorinha Squats

No. 39 Leg and Lower Back Stretch

No. 18 Back Bridge Push-Ups

As you do 50 cocorinha squats, rotate your wrists. On the final squat, sit in position for the front leg (and lower back) stretch and do one full stretch for 5 deep breaths. Lie back and do 10 bridge push-ups. Roll up and do another 50 cocorinha squats, then continue the cycle for 7½ minutes. See if you can crank out 3 full cycles of exercises in that time.

■ *Legs, shoulders, and back workout*

No. 3 Cocorinha Squats

No. 20 No Cheat Bridge

If you are already warmed up, say from a 7½-minute aú normal workout, tag on this combination to give your spine a backward arch to complement the lateral stretch from the aú normals. Do 50 rapid cocorinha squats, then rest back on one hand and reach over for the no cheat bridge. Then press the other hand on the floor and do a no cheat bridge in the other direction. Immediately shoot up for another 50 squats and continue the cycle.

The Next Stage

Hopefully you are beginning to see a pattern here. The 7½-minute workouts are a wake-up call for the body. If you tend toward a sedentary lifestyle, why not break up your day with two or three of these 7½-minute sessions? If you know you are going to spend six or seven hours at the computer, it's not so unrealistic to spend a small fraction of that time doing capoeira conditioning; or a few minutes before breakfast, a few in the evening. If you're worried about sweating, familiarize yourself with the "meia lua" wash. Hit the restroom, and a quick upper-body wash with soap and water takes only a couple of minutes and will get rid of any sweat you might build up during a 7½-minute workout.

The key is to combine the exercises so that every day you bend the spine forward, backward, and laterally. Also, try to give your legs some training, as leg strength and endurance are "the guvnors" in capoeira (as they say in England). The point is to work the muscles and mobilize the heart and lungs into action. Remember a muscle that doesn't work atrophies, so any amount of training, even as minimal as 7½-minutes, is insurance against the process of atrophying and acts as a toner for your whole system.

It is interesting to experiment with training. You may use these 7½-minute sessions, based as they are on variations of the cocorinha squat, mixed with other exercises, to try capoeira conditioning as an anaerobic training session.

Anaerobic Training

Anaerobic means "without oxygen." It is short bursts of much-increased exertion followed by a period of rest. The difference is that in capoeira conditioning, while you "rest," you do another set of exercises, working a different body part while you recover from your "oxygen debt." Oxygen debt is a situation in which the hard-working muscle tissues need more oxygen than they have available, resulting in a "debt" of oxygen and anaerobic respiration. Generally speaking, during anaerobic exercise you burn glycogen, which is sugar converted from carbohydrates. Anaerobic exercise—as in, for example, 50 rapid-fire cocorinha squats (No. 3) or aú normal (No. 25)—will raise your basal metabolism, and it will remain raised for a considerable period of time after you have finished exercising, thus burning more calories even when you are back at your desk.

If you have trained anaerobically and are in oxygen debt, you may need to inhale through your mouth briefly, yet try to bring your breathing back under control and begin nasal breathing as you recover during a new stage of the exercise cycle—for example, while you do no cheat back bridges (No. 20) or a bananeira handstand (No. 33).

Training Game: "Capoeira Fartlek"

Fartlek means "speed play" and was a running concept developed in Scandinavia in the 1930s. This type of training combines aerobic exercise (for example, long, steady distance running) with anaerobic exercise (speed surges of high intensity or hill sprints within the run). The fartlek effect can easily be utilized in capoeira conditioning. Take a set of 250 cocorinha squats. At an aerobic pace you will be able to build up to this number in 7½ minutes. But let's say you try to do 250 cocorinha squats in 6½ or 7 minutes, by doing 50 or 75 of them at a vastly increased pace, thus forcing your body to work anaerobically. There it is, "capoeira fartlek." You can use this speed play in any way you want during capoeira conditioning to work your body in a way that puts you in the "excessive post-exercise oxygen consumption" (EPOC) condition described earlier. Be imaginative, as variety keeps the training interesting and playful. Remember that we're doing this to stay fit, get healthy, feel good, and have fun, not to add burdens to our cares, and cares to our woes.

Naturally this is excellent training for the game of capoeira itself, where a change of gear is often called for inside the roda, and if you've done it in training, you are that much fitter to do it in the jogo.

Aerobic Training

Aerobic means "with oxygen." Dr. Kenneth H. Cooper popularized aerobic exercise after he published his book *Aerobics* in 1968. Almost any exercise can be done either anaerobically or aerobically. Capoeira conditioning is no exception. If you do these exercises at a sustainable, steady pace, increasing your heart rate without entering oxygen debt, you are doing an aerobic exercise.

The benefits of aerobic exercise are well known and manifest (but it will not hurt to recount them). You will gain improvements to your looks, your skin tone and glow. There will be increased oxygen consumption and blood volume, and lower blood pressure.

Your heart will work less with a lower resting heart rate. Aerobic training will fend off depression, and will release stress and tension, reducing anxiety as you produce endorphins. Endorphins are the natural pain-killing hormones produced by your body during sustained exercise. They give you a natural high and a feeling of well-being.

15-Minute Capoeira Conditioning Aerobic Sessions

Try the following combination suggestions, or build your own sessions. Because of the nature of capoeira, almost any of the movements will fit together as snugly as two adjoining jigsaw pieces. So be flexible and try a full range of exercises from those demonstrated within this book. To link exercises together, just do a No. 4 ginga in between movements to change your foot position.

Leg and aerobic workout

No. 3 Cocorinha Squats

Do 500 in 15 minutes.

Waist, legs, abs, shoulders, wrists, and back workout

No. 5 Ginga Reverse Waist Twist

No. 3 Cocorinha Squat

No. 41 Bênção

Ginga with the reverse twist by bringing one leg back. Return the foot to the middle parallel position again and cocorinha. Ginga back on the same foot, then bênção. Take the foot back again. Ginga and do the same thing on the other side. Do 100 to 150 in 7½ minutes. Then:

No. 9 Static Cabeçada

No. 21 Wall Wheel Bridge

Alternate these two movements for 7½ minutes.

Leg, waist, arms, and shoulders workout

No. 4 Ginga

No. 29 Negativa Lateral

Ginga for 10 steps. Negativa lateral to the right. Ginga for 10 steps and negativa lateral to the left. Repeat for 15 minutes.

Leg, waist, arms, shoulders, and back workout

No. 4 Ginga

No. 30/31 Moenda

Ginga for 10 steps, then moenda to the right, ginga, and moenda to the left. Repeat for 15 minutes.

Legs, arms, shoulders, and waist workout

No. 28 Aú Pistols

Side to side, try to do as many reps of the pistols as you can between aús. As you tire, simply lower the number of reps you do each set. Repeat for 15 minutes, resting with No. 4 ginga.

Legs, arms, shoulders, back, and hips workout

No. 1 Cocorinha

No. 9 Static Cabeçada

No. 32 Queda de Quatro-Chapa

No. 20 No Cheat Bridge

Assume No. 1 cocorinha. Shoot forward for a No. 9 static cabeçada, then back into No. 1 cocorinha and immediately drop into No. 32 queda de quatro-chapa (both left and right legs). Finish with No. 20 no cheat back bridge to right and left. Repeat the sequence as many times as you can in 15 minutes.

Chest, legs, back, and shoulders workout

No. 37 Leg Stretch Push-Ups

No. 18 Back Bridge Push-Ups

No. 38 Side Split Twists

Do a set of No. 37 leg stretch push-ups, then a set of back bridge push-ups. Recover your breath while "resting" in a set of No. 38 side split twists. Repeat process for 15 minutes.

30-, 45-, and 60-Minute Capoeira Conditioning Sessions

If you are feeling full of energy and have the time to spare, you can try a longer session once in a while, maybe once or twice a week.

By now you will already be familiar with the exercises and have built up a core of capoeira strength and conditioning, so you will be in a position to choose which exercises you want to put together.

In this case, it will probably be best to suggest principles rather than set workouts.

Try, at least once or twice a week, to include a good solid session of some variation of the four basic core movements (No. 3 cocorinha squats, No. 14 back bridge, No. 25 aú normal, and No.

33/34 plantanda bananeira and bananeira push-up). By including these within your overall capoeira conditioning program, you will ensure your body has the inner strength to perform all the other capoeira movements.

Mentally, or even on a piece of paper, break your body down into parts and arrange exercise sessions so that you don't neglect any part of your frame. There's little benefit to developing shoulders like an Olympic gymnast if you have the legs of a sparrow.

Ginga is a good warm-up exercise. It's a dance step, so you can do it to music for 10 or 15 minutes or so. Added to cocorinha squats it will give the legs a powerful boost whenever you do it. Keep in mind the capoeira principle of the hands being feet and the feet being hands.

Devote at least 50 percent of your training to exercises on your hands. That includes all the bananeira exercises, the aú movements, the negativa lateral, the bridges, and so on.

Think of your spine often and devote whole sessions to looking after it. Bend forward, backward, to each side, and twist your spine.

Think aerobic. Keep it simple; take any two or three of these movements and put them together for half an hour and you've got a capoeira conditioning session.

One of the main de-motivators to training or beginning a course of exercise toward learning a "martial art" is to think you need a whole load of esoteric, "deep" knowledge to do it. You don't. To play capoeira well is a long process that demands lots of practice with other capoeira players for sure. Yet to get in great shape using capoeira movements you don't need any esoteric knowledge at all. Just the get-up-and-go to devote a minimum of 15 minutes a day to performing these exercises with good form and strong mental focus.

Chapter 3

The Exercises

For a quick reference guide and to help you make a "no-brainer" decision on what to do for a desired result in any particular workout, each exercise is accompanied by some buzzwords that describe what it is mostly effective for. The buzzwords are:

1. **Flexibility-stretch**
2. **Strength**
3. **Power**
4. **Agility**
5. **Balance**
6. **Cardio (cardiovascular endurance)**
7. **Coordination**
8. **Fat Burner**

Please note that "fat burning" isn't a quality of overall fitness in itself; therefore, it wasn't in the initial list of essential attributes for all-around conditioning. Fat burning, though, ***is*** an attribute of some of these exercises, and is included here for those who have a particular interest in losing some weight.

Below is a very simple chart so you can go straight to the exercises that best achieve the result you want. For example, you want to burn fat and build strength today. Just check out the "Fat Burner" and "Strength" boxes below and go to the exercises corresponding to the numbers within each box. If you want more details on what those exercises do for you—for instance, what part of your body they will strengthen, and so forth—you can then read the "Health and Fitness Benefits" section within each exercise description.

Note that core movements are in parentheses.

Training Effects Chart

This Training Effects Chart will guide you to particular exercises that emphasize different areas of overall conditioning. Exercises that relate to core movements will be shown in bold print and in parentheses. If numbers other than the core movements (**3**), (**14**), (**25**), (**33**), and (**34**) are shown in bold print, it is because they are exercises closely related to the core movements, which work similar areas of conditioning, though with a slightly different emphasis.

Training Effects Chart

Effect	**Exercise Numbers**
Flexibility-stretch	1, 2, (**3**), 5, 6, 7, 8, 10, 11, 12, 13, (**14**), (**15**), 16, 17, (**18**), 19, 20, 21, 22, 23, 24, (**25**), 26, 27, 28, 29, 30, 31, 32, 35, 37, 38, 39
Strength	9, (**14**), (**15**), 16, 17, (**18**), 19, 20, 21, 22, 24, (**25**), 26, 27, 28, 29, 30, 31, (**33**), (**34**), 35, 36, 37, 40
Power	(**3**), 7, (**18**), 19, 28, (**34**)
Agility	4, 5, 6, 7, (**25**), 26, 30, 31, (**34**)
Balance	4, 9, 17, (**18**), 19, 20, 21, 22, 23, 24, (**25**), 26, 27, 28, 29, (**33**), (**34**), 35, 36
Cardio (cardiovascular endurance)	(**3**), 4, 5, 6, 7, (**18**), 22, (**25**), 26, 27, 28, 40
Fat Burner	(**3**), 4, 5, 6, 7, (**25**), 26, 28, 40
Coordination	4, 5, 6, 7, 20, 22, (**25**), 26, 28, 30, 31

1. Cocorinha (stationary)

Flexibility-stretch.

Movement

Stand with your feet shoulder-width (at least 15 to 20 inches) apart. Bend your knees and drop down into a squat position with your hands in front of you, crossed at the wrist.

Breathing

Breathe deeply. Try nasal breathing, inhaling and exhaling only through your nose. Exhale until you feel you have expelled every last breath of air from your lungs, and as you exhale, visualize your lower spine (sacroiliac joint) relaxing farther toward the floor. Hold the cocorinha position for at least eight breaths.

Pointers

If you have stiff ankles, squat in the same way, but with your heels raised on a couple of thin books, weight-training plates, or even a rolled-up towel.

Health and Fitness Benefits

This is very beneficial for the sacroiliac joints at the back of the pelvis and base of the spine. It releases pressure on your lower back, lowers the sacrum between the hip joints, and gives the ankles a powerful stretch.

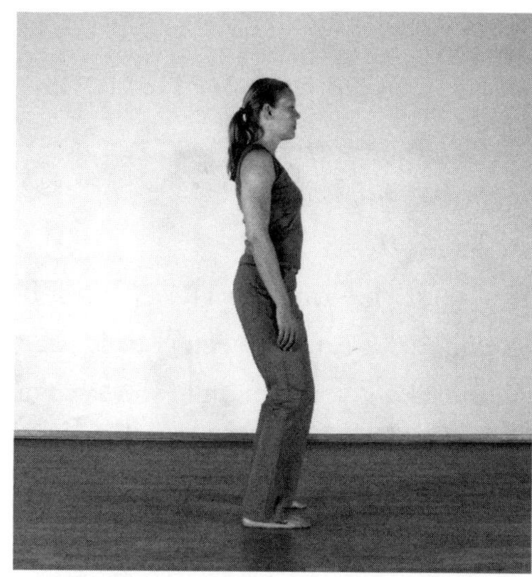

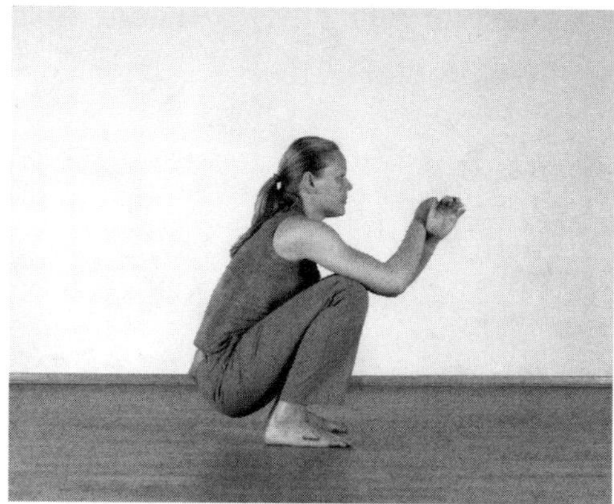

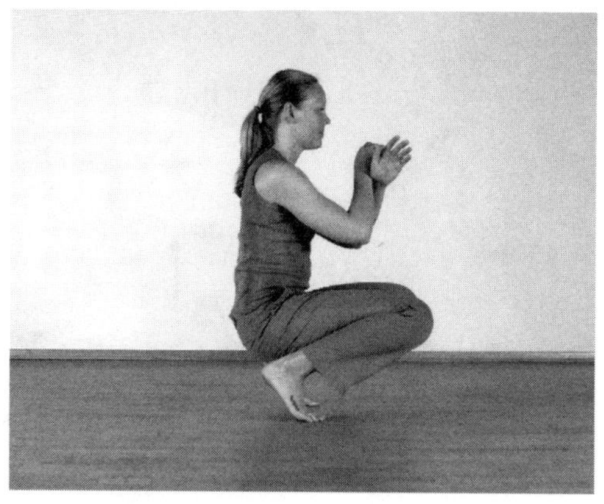

2. Cocorinha Variations

Flexibility-stretch.

Movement

Rest your chin on your chest for a fuller stretch of the spine and let your arms rest between your legs.

Outstretch your arms and squeeze your shoulder blades together, lifting your chin for an opposite stretch. You can have your heels flat on the ground, or if you prefer, raised as they are in the photograph.

If your ankles and legs are so stiff that you find it difficult to balance without falling over backward, hold a secure table leg or other secure object for stability.

Breathing

As for cocorinha.

Pointers

Once again, let your tailbone drop low. While you hold onto an object for stability you can rotate around slightly and work on releasing tension in your lower spine.

Health and Fitness Benefits

Similar to those for cocorinha.

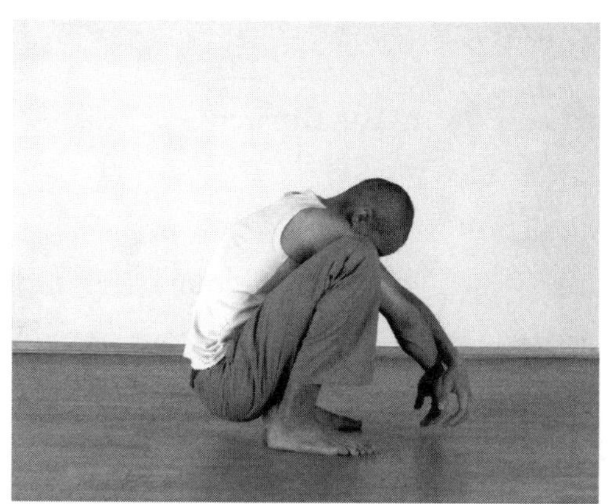

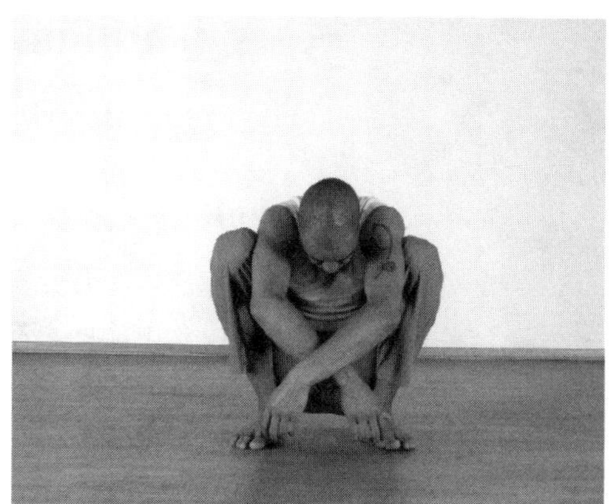

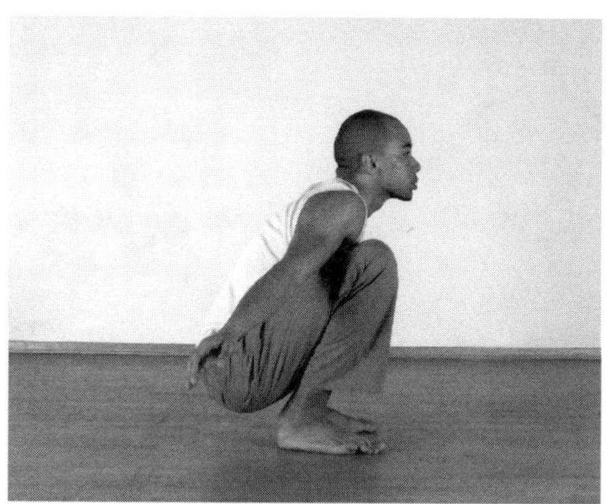

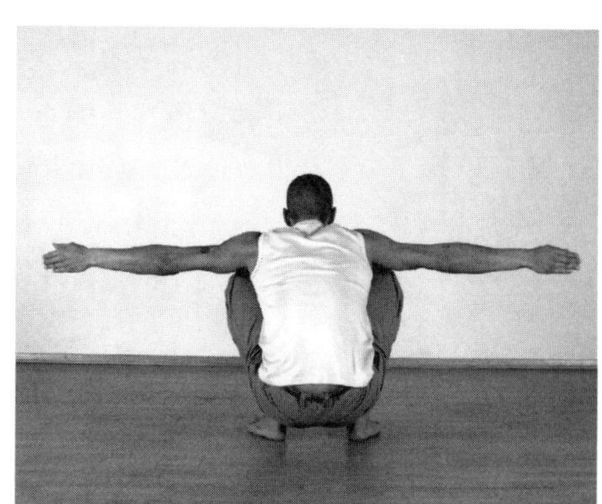

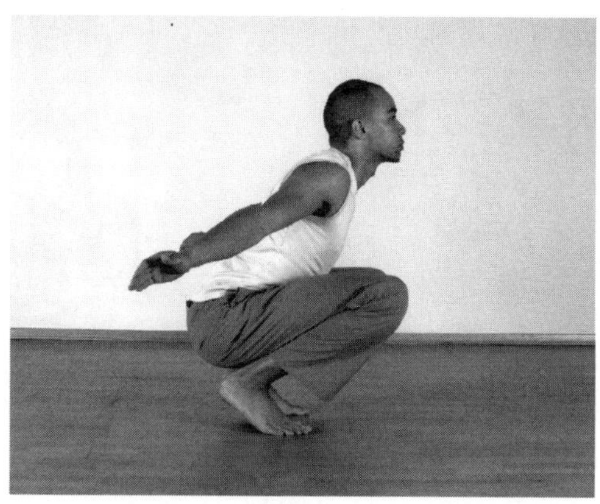

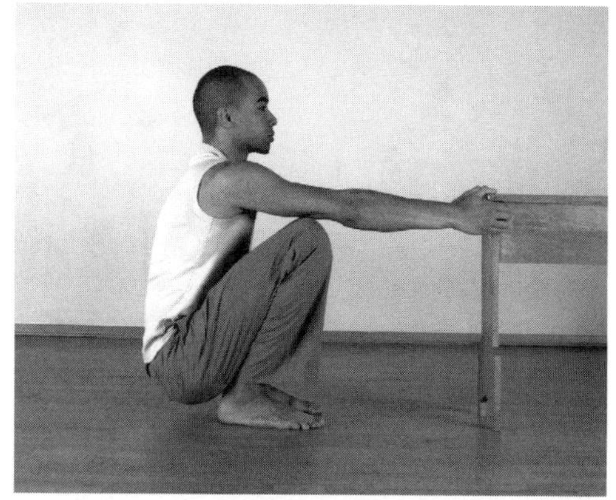

3. Cocorinha (squat)

Flexibility-stretch. Cardio. Power. Fat Burner.

Movement

Stand with your feet shoulder-width apart. Bend your knees and drop down into a squat position with your hands in front of you, crossed at the wrist. Stand up again, bringing your arms above your head and reaching toward the sky for a full stretch of the spine. Repeat. Shoot for 175 in 5 minutes, 350 in 10 minutes, or 500 in 15 minutes.

Breathing

Exhale on the way down. Inhale on the way up. In all exercises try nasal breathing, or if you find that difficult, inhale through the nose and exhale through the mouth.

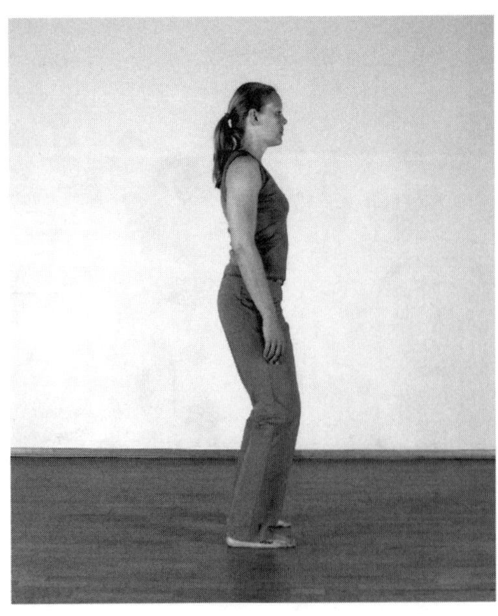

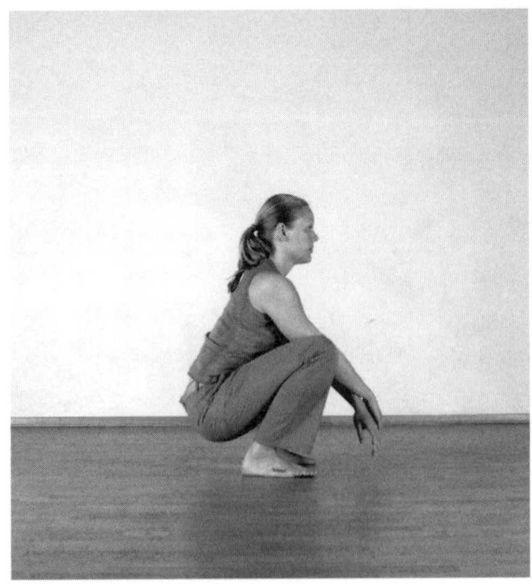

Pointers

Let your hips drop as low as possible. Try not to bend forward on the way down, or on the way up. Keep your head upright and aligned with your spine. If your ankles are not flexible enough to fully squat with your heels on the floor, you can raise your heels and squat on your toes.

Health and Fitness Benefits

If you do these squats rapidly and in high repetitions, they build incredible power and springiness into your legs. Aim to do a top number of 500 cocorinha squats in around 15 minutes and you will also be giving your cardiovascular system a very thorough work-out.

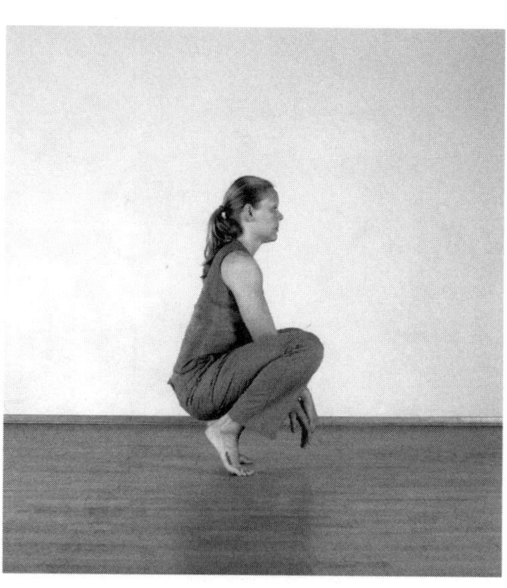

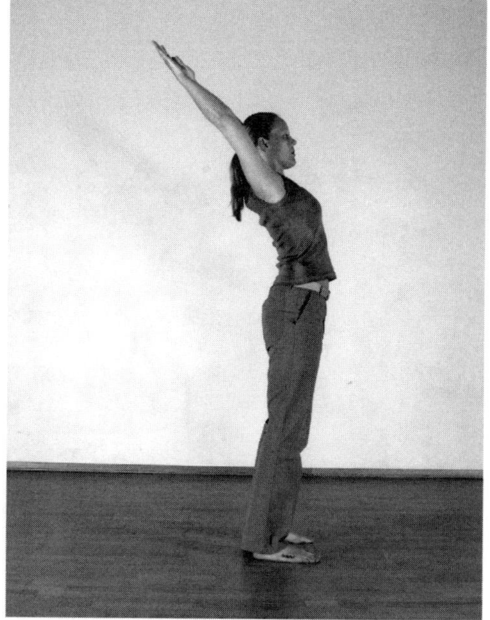

4. Ginga (basic capoeira footwork)

Agility. Coordination. Balance. Cardio. Fat Burner.

Movement

Stand with your feet shoulder-width apart with your knees slightly bent. Slide one leg back and rest most of your weight on the ball of your back foot, with the heel up. The sole of your front foot should be flat on the floor (both knees remain bent throughout the whole sequence). Simultaneously raise your arm and hand and swing it to the front of your face or chest on the same side as your back leg.

Transfer your weight back to the front foot, simultaneously sliding the back foot to its original parallel position. Switch arms and legs so that your other foot slides back and your other arm swings up in front of your body.

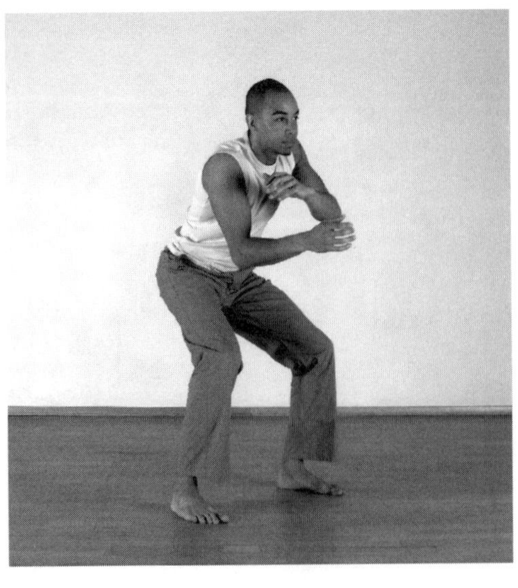

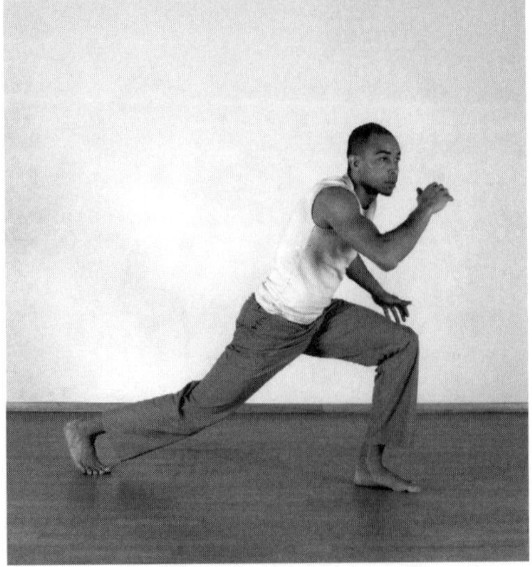

Breathing

Breathe freely.

Pointers

Don't drop the back heel. Be on the ball of the back foot. Lean forward slightly at all times in the ginga, and remember it's a dance step, so get into a rhythm and swing from side to side. "Gingar" is the verb "to swing" in Portuguese.

Don't straighten the front leg or raise the front toes when you do ginga. Note: The description says to slide your foot back; it doesn't have to keep contact with the floor, although it doesn't rise very high either, maybe just one or two inches.

Health and Fitness Benefits

This is a great exercise for balance and coordination. If you do it to music, try various tempos; at a faster rhythm it is a good aerobic exercise.

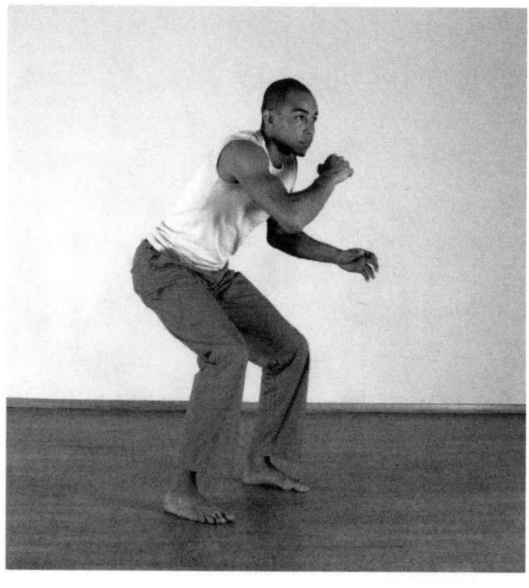

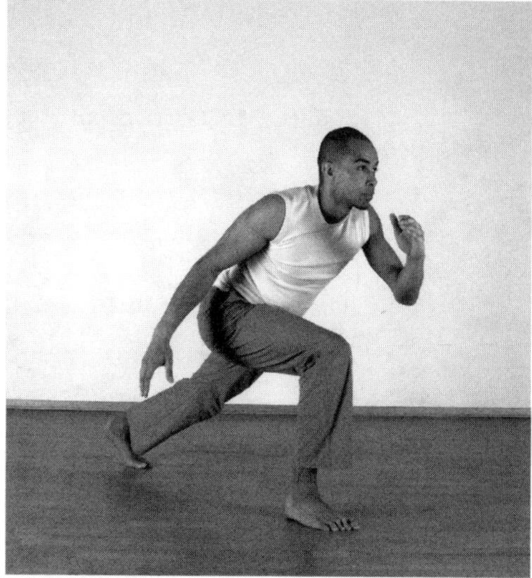

5. Ginga with a Reverse Twist at the Waist

Flexibility-stretch. Coordination. Agility. Cardio. Fat Burner.

Movement

Do ginga in a similar way to the regular movement, except when your weight is on the ball of the back right foot, twist at the waist to your left, taking your left arm straight out behind you and looking over your left shoulder.

Stay in this position for a beat and then shift back to the frontal position, swap legs as in regular ginga, and when your left foot is fully extended back, twist to the right in the same way, right arm extended behind you and looking over your right shoulder.

Breathing

Breathe freely.

Pointers

Twist fully and try to reach back and rotate your waist, spine, and neck as far as you can for maximum benefit. Imagine you are wringing water from a towel as you twist your waist.

Health and Fitness Benefits

This rotation of your spine and neck loosens you up for many capoeira movements, helping to maintain mobility and fluidity the whole length of your back.

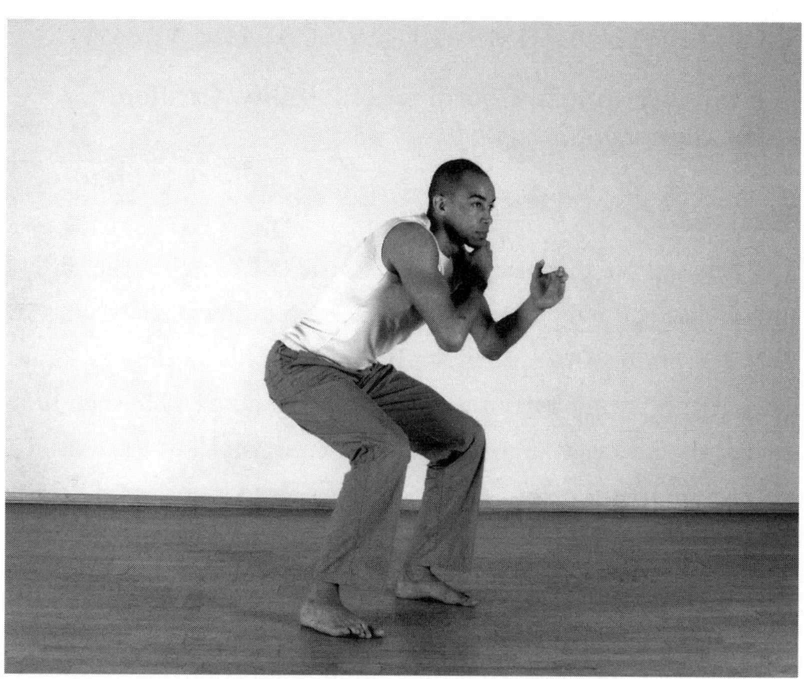

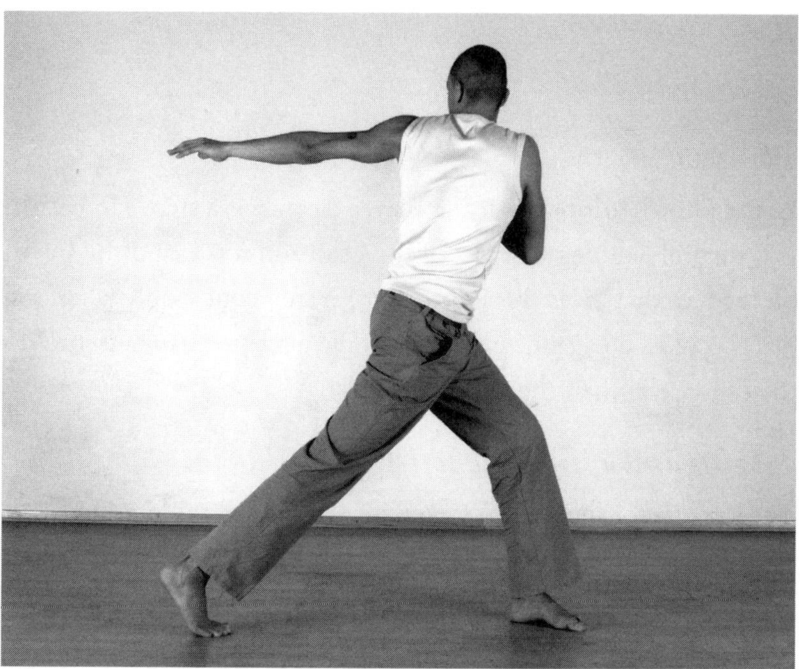

6. Ginga with a Full Twist at the Waist

Flexibility-stretch. Coordination. Agility. Cardio. Fat Burner.

Movement

This is based on a similar principle to the last exercise; the difference is that you twist toward your back leg rather than away from it. In the photo, the capoeirista begins with his left leg back and straight and right leg front and bent (as in a ginga). He then fully rotates first his head, then shoulders, then waist, all to the left, in a 360-degree rotation, and swivels on his feet, so that his right leg is straightened and left leg bent. He ends up looking to the front again, having rotated as far as he can without taking a step. Then come back to the original position, do one ginga to change feet, and repeat the movement in the opposite direction.

Breathing

Breathe freely.

Pointers

In the photo, it looks as if the player has taken a step. He hasn't. It is the full 360-degree twist of the head and torso, and the swivel on the feet that gives this impression. A step comes only when the player centers up again, and does a single ginga to change feet to do the exercise in the other direction.

Health and Fitness Benefits

The same as for the previous exercise. This is a good mobility exercise, giving an excellent spinal twist and increasing lightness and agility on the balls of the feet.

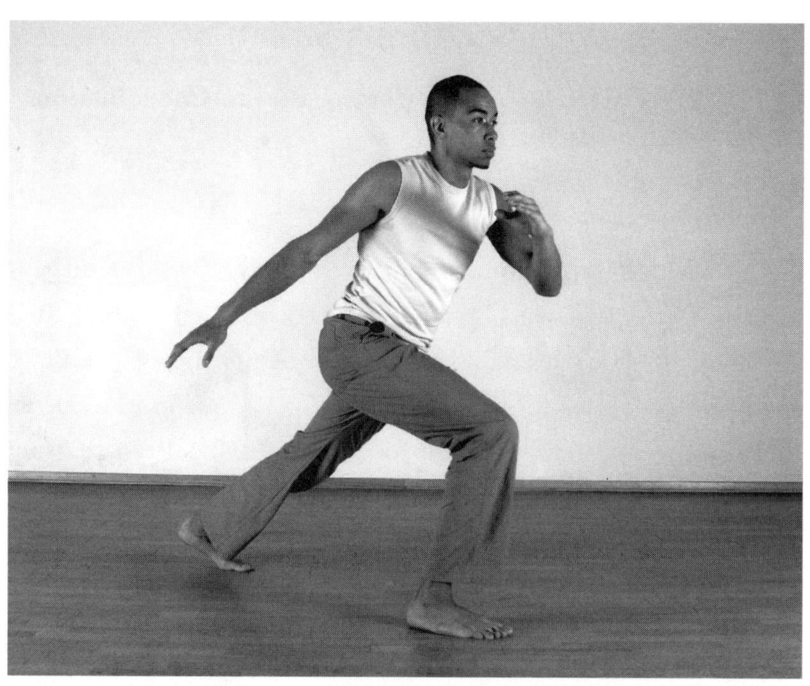

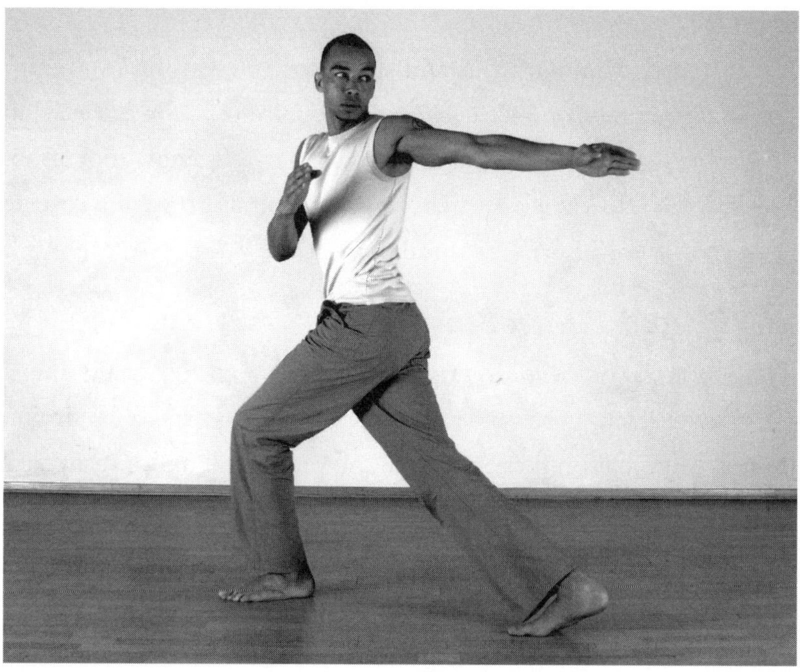

7. Ginga with Cocorinha Squat

Flexibility-stretch. Agility. Cardio. Power. Coordination. Accelerated Fat Burner.

Movement

In this tough exercise you combine No. 3 and No. 4 together for a very effective workout. Begin in basic cocorinha position and as you come up slide your right leg back into a ginga movement. Once the right leg comes forward and parallel again, drop into cocorinha. Spring up, sliding the left foot to the back. Alternate using ginga from side to side with a cocorinha in the middle position.

Breathing

Try nasal breathing: exhale on the way down, and inhale on the way up.

Pointers

Get into a rhythm with this and shoot for 100 reps in 5 minutes, 200 in 10 minutes, or 300 (even more if you're very conditioned) in 15 minutes. Count each drop into cocorinha as a single repetition. You can also do the cocorinha-ginga combination with a reverse twist (No. 5) or ginga with a full twist at the waist (No. 6).

Health and Fitness Benefits

This is a fantastic conditioning workout for your heart and lungs, your lower back, your ankles, your spine, and your thighs. If you do this combination for 5, 10, or 15 minutes you'll find it really gets your heart pumping and works up a sweat.

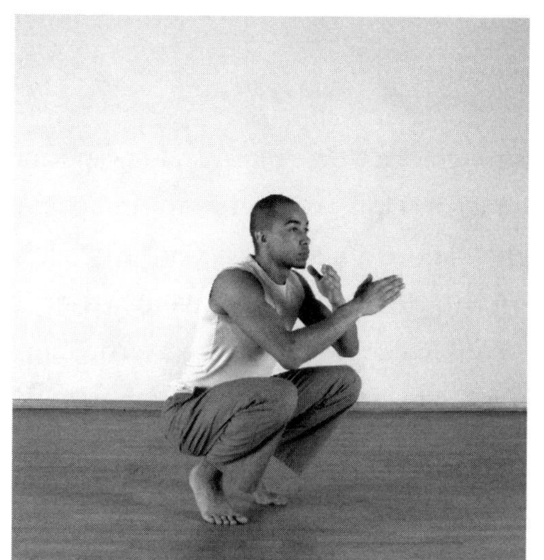
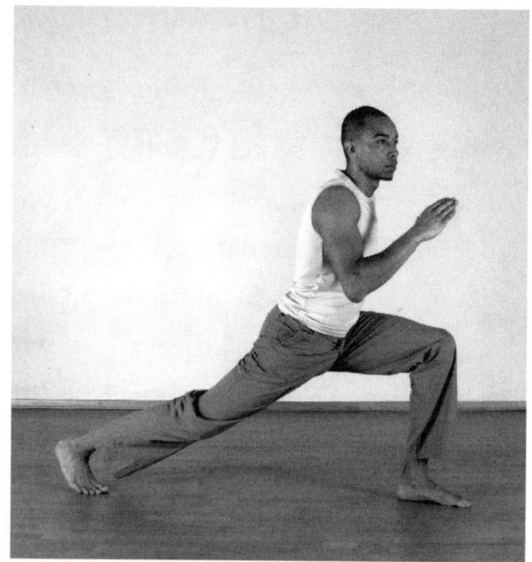
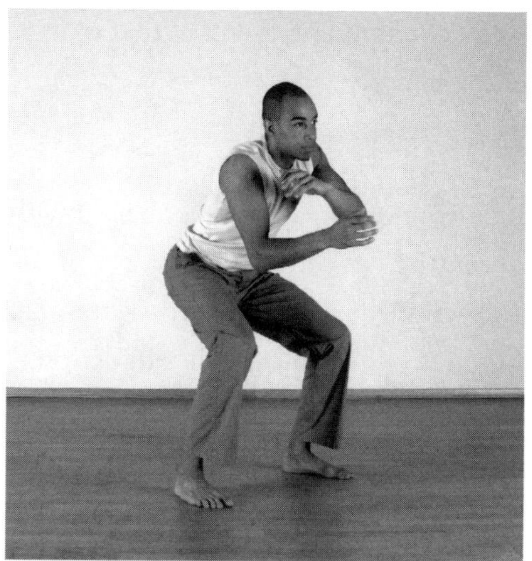
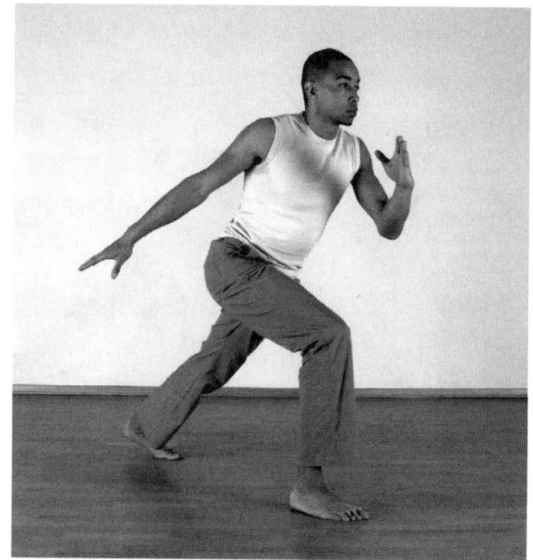

8. Wrist Rotation

Flexibility-stretch.

Note: Your body is only as strong as its weakest link, and in capoeira that weakest link is often the wrist. Don't neglect to warm up and stretch your wrists thoroughly before doing bridges or cartwheels ("aú" in capoeira). It is better to exert pressure on your wrists in a graded, steady way than to immediately launch into a jarring aú-type movement or a bananeira, which may create a glitch in your wrist that will spoil your workout.

Even experienced capoeiristas sometimes find that after one movement with the weight on their hands, one wrist is giving them pain. Therefore, do some of these wrist warm-ups every time you play capoeira or do any capoeira conditioning exercises that require you to hold your weight on the hands.

Movement

Hold your arms straight out in front of you at shoulder height with the wrists bent and fingers pointing upward. Rotate wrists so the fingers move inward, then downward, then outward. Rotate 25 times in this direction, and then 25 times in the other direction.

Breathing

Breathe freely.

Pointers

You may find that your shoulders, forearms, and wrists become fatigued by doing the recommended 50 reps total. Persevere and try to focus on putting the wrists through the fullest range of movement. If you get tired, slow down, breathe deeply, and try to relax your shoulders as you rotate your wrists.

Health and Fitness Benefits

Wrist tension or movement restriction will impede capoeira proficiency and make certain movements (for instance, the bridge) more difficult. Mobility in the wrists will increase the mobility in your elbows and shoulders too. The warm-up will help prevent injury to the hands' nerves and tendons.

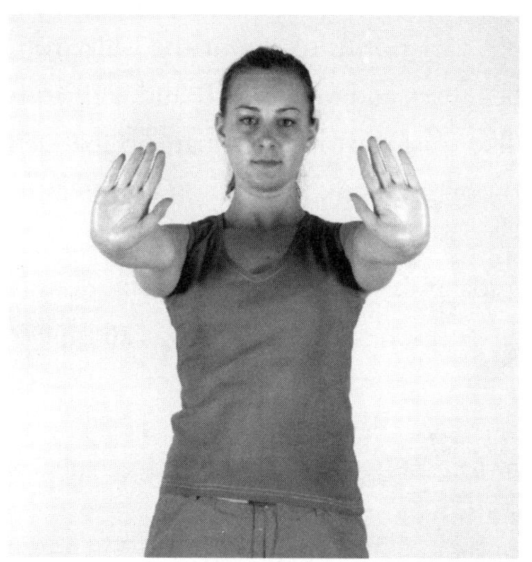

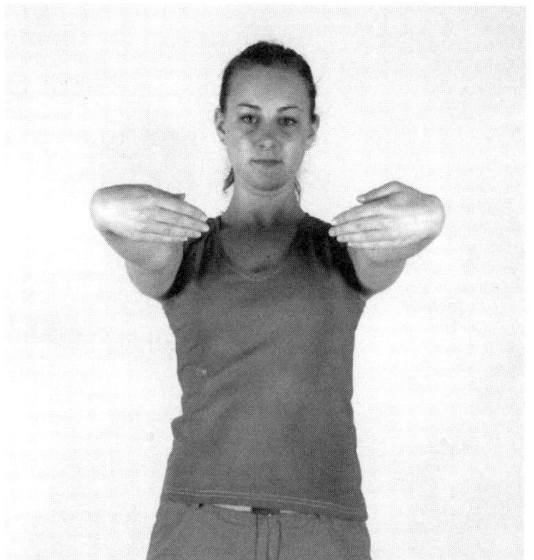

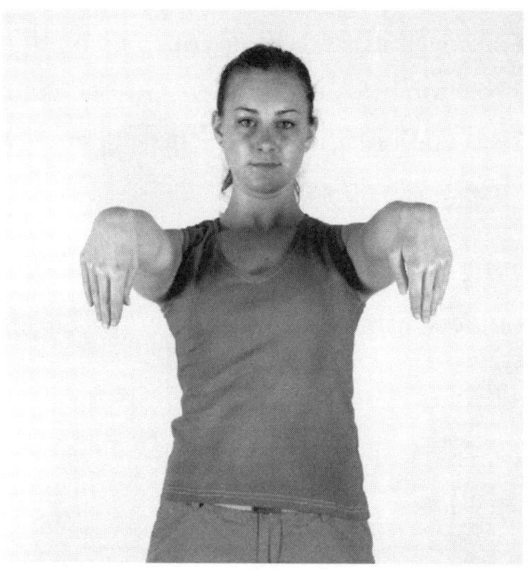

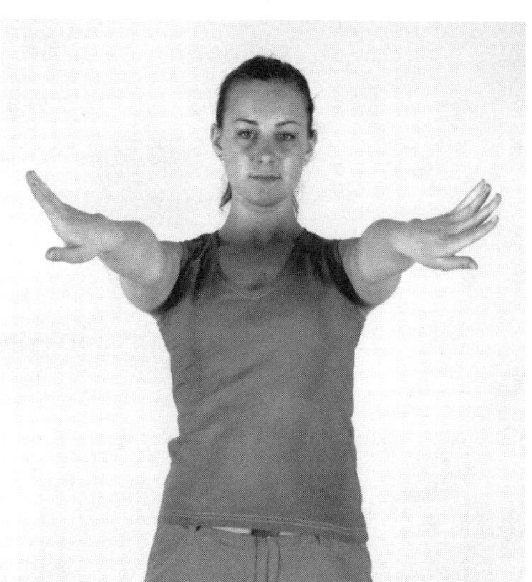

9. Cabeçada (static posture)

Balance. Strength.

Movement

Start in a cocorinha and lunge forward slowly, walking your hands into a static push-up position. Keep your head, spine, pelvis, and straight legs in alignment. A variation is to repeat the walk from cocorinha into static cabeçada, back and forth slowly and with control as many times as you like. Just start in the squat, tip forward placing your palms on the floor, and walk forward on your hands, keeping the balls of the feet where they are. Then when the body is fully extended in the cabeçada, walk back on the hands and resume the original cocorinha squat position. Repeat 10, 20, or 30 times.

Breathing

Once you are in position try to take between 6 and 10 deep inhalations and exhalations through the nose.

Pointers

Try not to sag at the waist. As well as stretching your wrists, this will give you a powerful contraction in your shoulders. Stretch your fingers wide and concentrate as you breathe; feel the flow of energy down your arms into your hands as you exhale.

Health and Fitness Benefits

Builds strength in your shoulders, arms, and wrists.

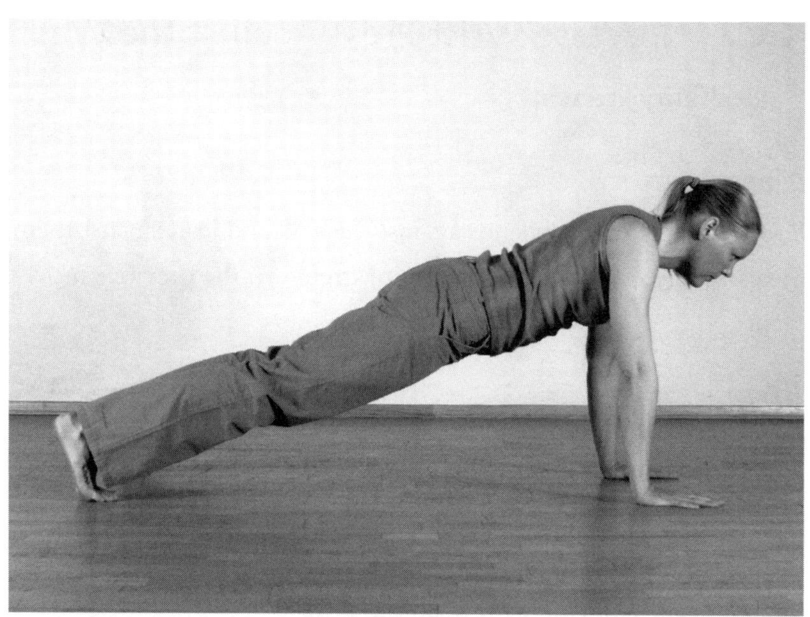

10. Reverse Wrist Press Against the Wall

Flexibility-stretch.

Movement

Place the back of your hands against the wall and lean against them with straight arms to get an opposite stretch to the previous movement.

Breathing

Similar to No. 9.

Pointers

Keep your arms straight and get an increased stretch by raising the level of your hands upward from the floor.

Health and Fitness Benefits

As in No. 8.

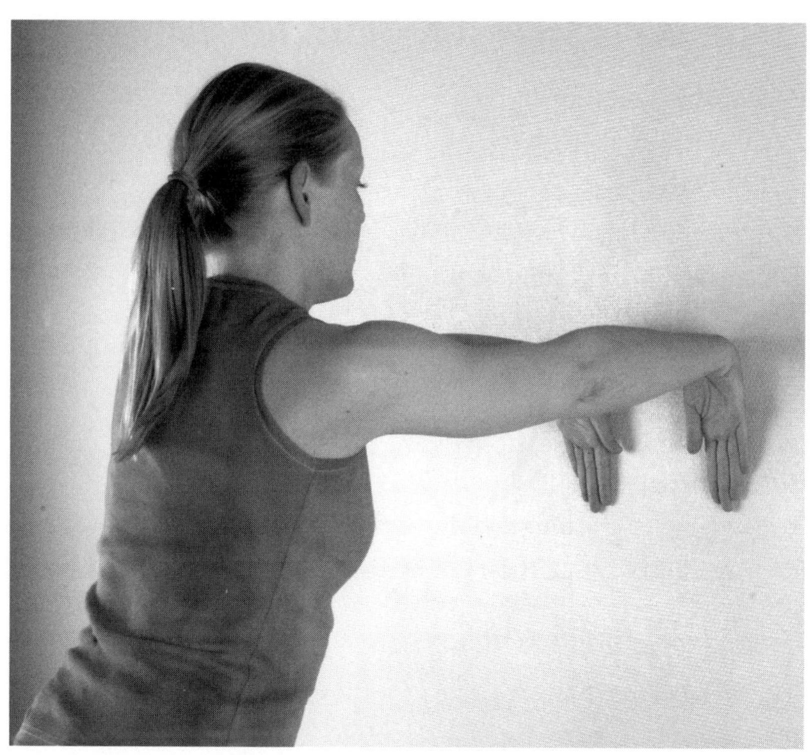

11. Wrist Stretch Against the Wall

Flexibility-stretch.

Movement

Stand leaning against the wall with your arms straight and palms flat against the wall, fingers pointing upward.

Breathing

Similar to No. 9.

Pointers

By lowering your hands and the angle of your arms you will increase the angle of the stretch on your wrist.

Health and Fitness Benefits

The benefits are those described for the other wrist-mobility movements.

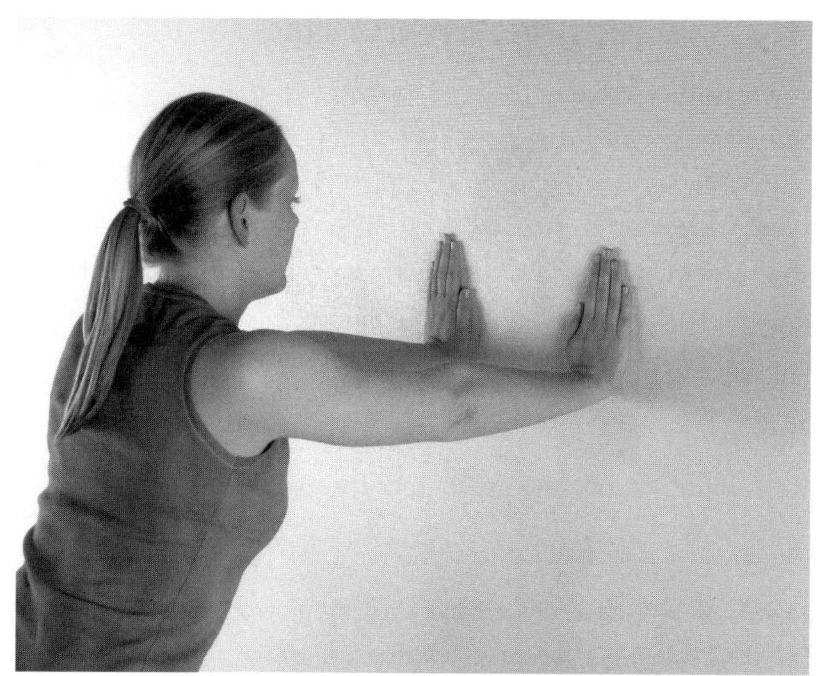

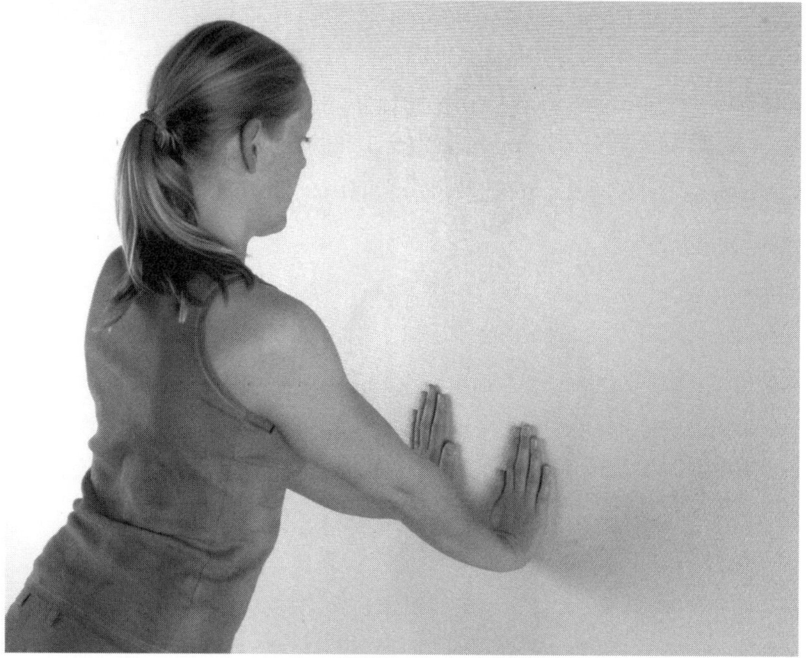

12. Basic Bridge Warm-Up

Flexibility-stretch.

Movement

Stand with your back to a wall, arch your back, and stretch your arms upward and backward so that the palms of your hands touch the wall when your arms are straight. Keep your feet flat on the floor, parallel, and approximately shoulder-width apart.

Breathing

Six deep inhalations and exhalations through the nostrils.

Pointers

Make sure you stand neither too far from nor too close to the wall. Position yourself so you can comfortably reach the wall and perform a full stretch with your straight arms back. Look back at the wall for a full stretch from the base of your spine to your neck.

Health and Fitness Benefits

Backward bending compresses the spinal vertebrae and will expand your abdomen and chest, which in turn enables you to breathe more deeply.

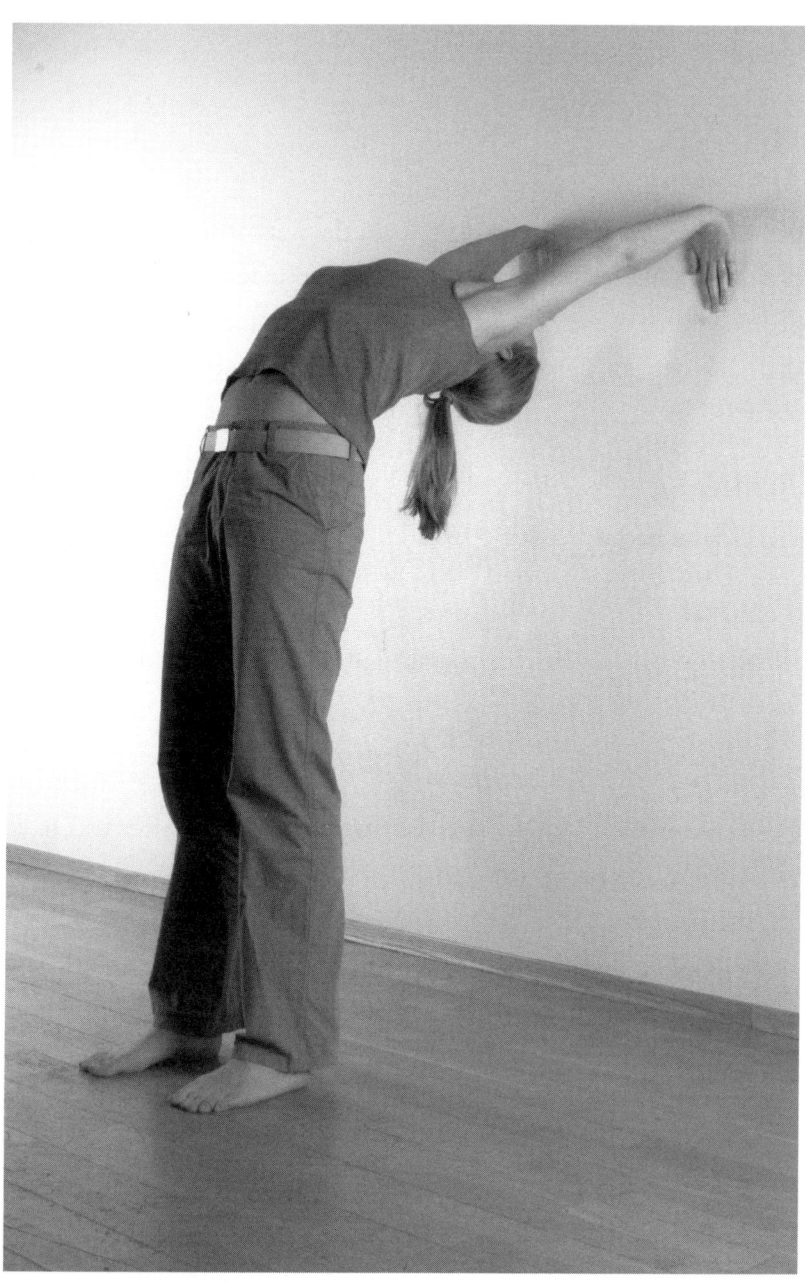

13. Basic Forward Bend

Flexibility-stretch.

Movement

Stand upright and bend forward from the waist, touching the palms of your hands on the floor in front of your feet, if possible. For people with stiff legs, keep them slightly bent and feel the stretch at the back of your pelvis. If you are supple, keep the knees straight for a full stretch.

Breathing

Deep nasal breathing for 6 breaths.

Pointers

When you exhale, allow your head and shoulders to drop downward toward your feet.

Health and Fitness Benefits

Forward bending is important for full spinal fitness. After you have been doing any backward spinal bending movements (such as No. 12, the basic bridge warm-up) it is a good idea to do a basic forward bend for balance and to release and lengthen the spine. The forward bend with straight legs will also stretch your hamstrings for greater flexibility in your legs. Holding the position and breathing will tone your waist and bring elasticity to your spine.

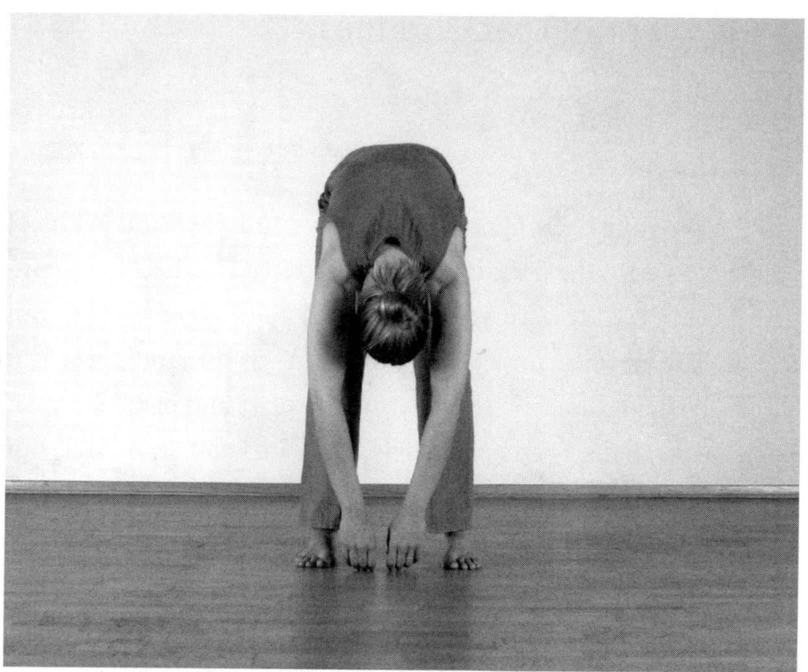

14. Ponte (back bridge)

Flexibility-stretch. Strength.

Movement

Lie flat on your back. Raise your elbows and press the palms of your hands onto the floor by your ears, so that the tips of your fingers are directed toward your feet. Bend your knees so that your feet are drawn up against your buttocks. Your feet and lower legs should be approximately shoulder-width apart and parallel.

As you exhale, raise your pelvis and torso and straighten out your arms so that your head rises from the floor, arms straight. In the full version, the soles of your feet remain flat on the floor.

To come out of the bridge bring your chin to your chest and slowly lower yourself onto your shoulders, then lie flat, or roll up onto your feet into a cocorinha.

Breathing

While holding the bridge, breathe deeply through the nose. Try for 3, 6, or 10 full, deep breaths. Always focus on breathing while you are bridging. If you are stiff and hold your breath or try to force the movement, it will make it more difficult.

Pointers

If you are on a slippery floor and either your hands or your feet keep slipping, try wearing thin rubber-soled shoes and wet the palms of your hands slightly so they don't slip. Relax your head so it drops down naturally between your arms.

Health and Fitness Benefits

The back bridge gives a strong stretch to the front of your body, and the spine is lengthened by the arch. This expands your chest and abdomen. The wrists and ankles are strengthened and the circulation is stimulated.

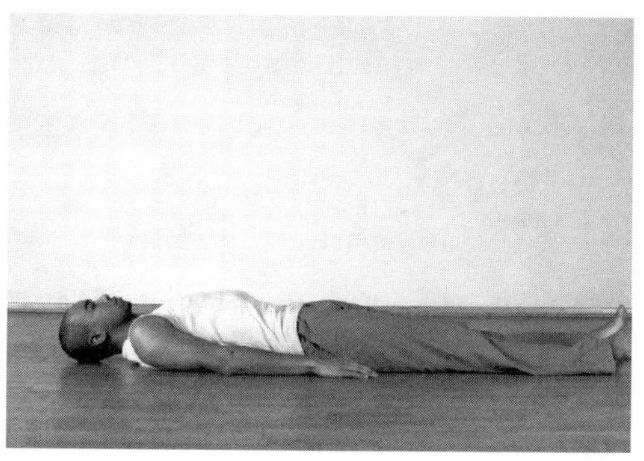

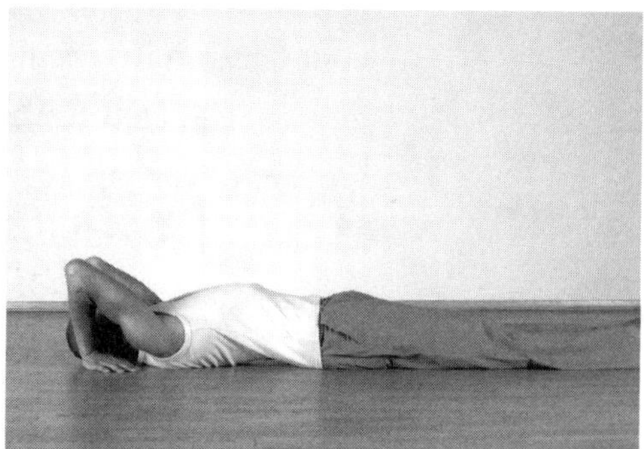

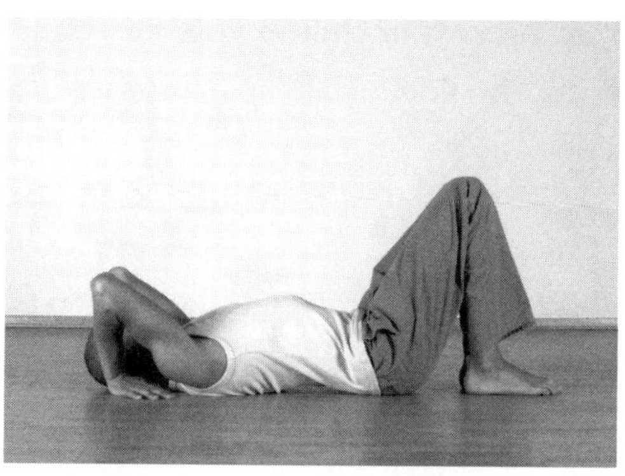

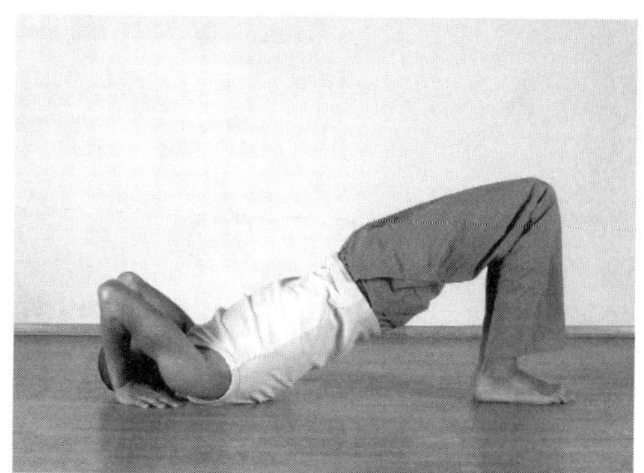

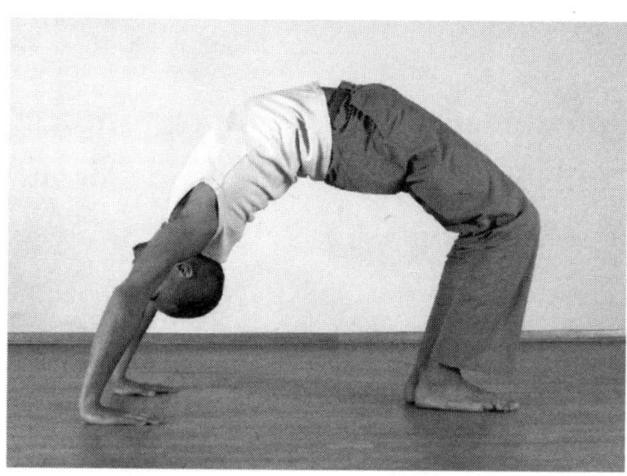

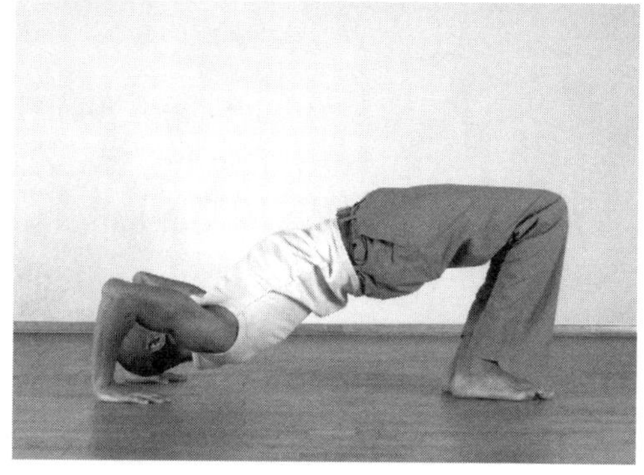

15. Back Bridge (heels raised)

Flexibility-stretch. Strength.

Movement

Lie flat on your back. Raise your elbows and press the palms of your hands onto the floor by your ears, so that the tips of your fingers are directed toward your feet. Bend your knees so that your feet are drawn up against your buttocks. Your feet and lower legs should be approximately shoulder-width apart and parallel.

As you exhale, raise your pelvis and torso and straighten out your arms so that your head rises from the floor, arms straight. In this (the easier) version, raise your heels and support yourself on the balls of your feet.

To come out of the bridge bring your chin to your chest and slowly lower yourself onto your shoulders, then lie flat, or roll up onto your feet into a cocorinha.

Breathing

While holding the bridge, breathe deeply through the nose. Try for 3, 6, or 10 full, deep breaths. Always focus on breathing while you are bridging. If you are stiff and hold your breath or try to force the movement, it will make it more difficult.

Pointers

If you are on a slippery floor and either your hands or your feet keep slipping, try wearing thin rubber-soled shoes and wet the palms of your hands slightly so they don't slip. Relax your head so it drops down naturally between your arms. This on-your-toes version is an easier option for people who are stiffer in their hips or shoulders.

Health and Fitness Benefits

The back bridge gives a strong stretch to the front of your body, and the spine is lengthened by the arch. This expands your chest and abdomen. The wrists and ankles are strengthened and the circulation is stimulated.

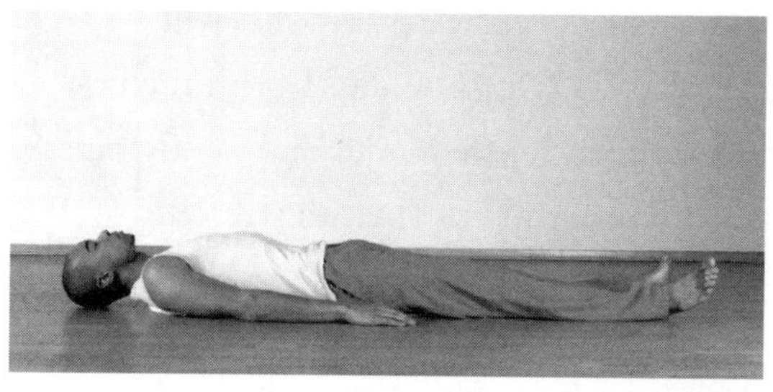

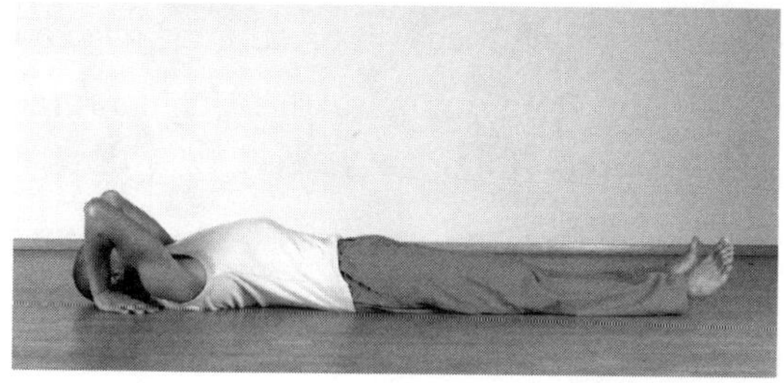

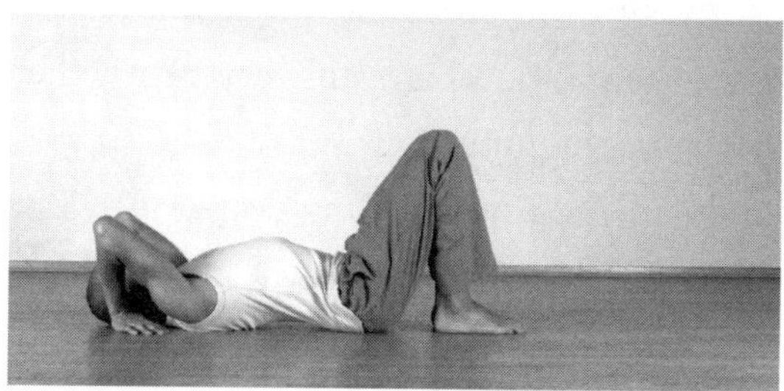

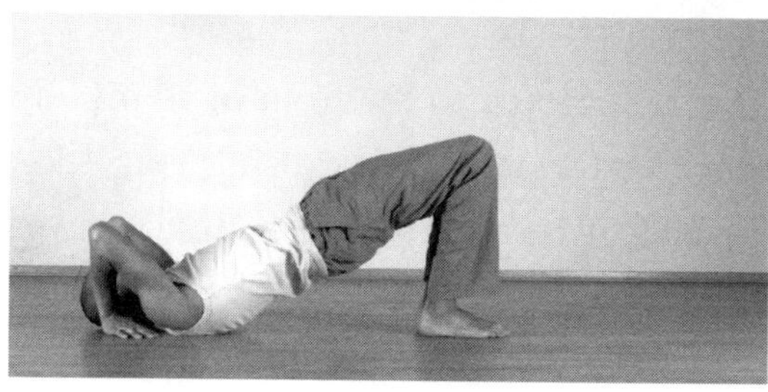

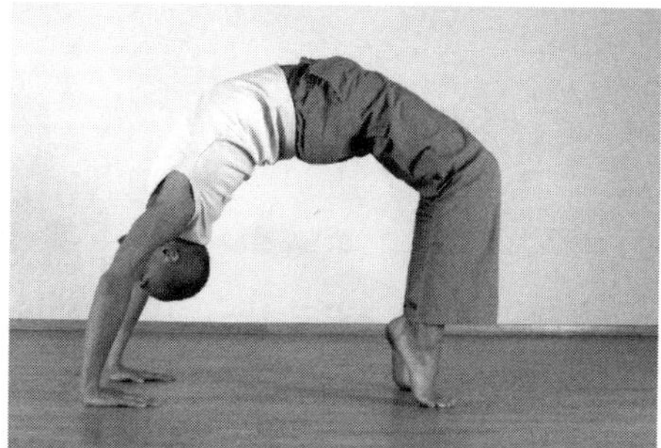

16. Back Bridge (assisted stretch)

Flexibility-stretch. Strength.

Movement

This is the same as for the basic bridge or the basic bridge on your toes. In this case you can work with a partner who will stand at your head; once you have reached your full length with the bridge, they put their hand under your shoulder blades and gently pull up to assist you in locking out your arms for the full stretch.

Breathing

While holding the bridge, breathe deeply through the nose. Try for 3, 6, or 10 full, deep breaths. Always focus on breathing while you are bridging. If you are stiff and hold your breath or try to force the movement, it will make it more difficult.

Pointers

The person supporting should not be pulling you up as if hoisting a heavy object. They assist your own effort and when you reach a sticking point (for instance, your elbows are still very bent), they gently pull to assist you in straightening them. If they hoist, they will merely lift your hands off the floor or drag you along. The assisted stretch can be done with heels up or down, though heels down gives you the longer stretch.

Health and Fitness Benefits

The back bridge gives a strong stretch to the front of your body, and the spine is lengthened by the arch. This expands your chest and abdomen. The wrists and ankles are strengthened and the circulation is stimulated.

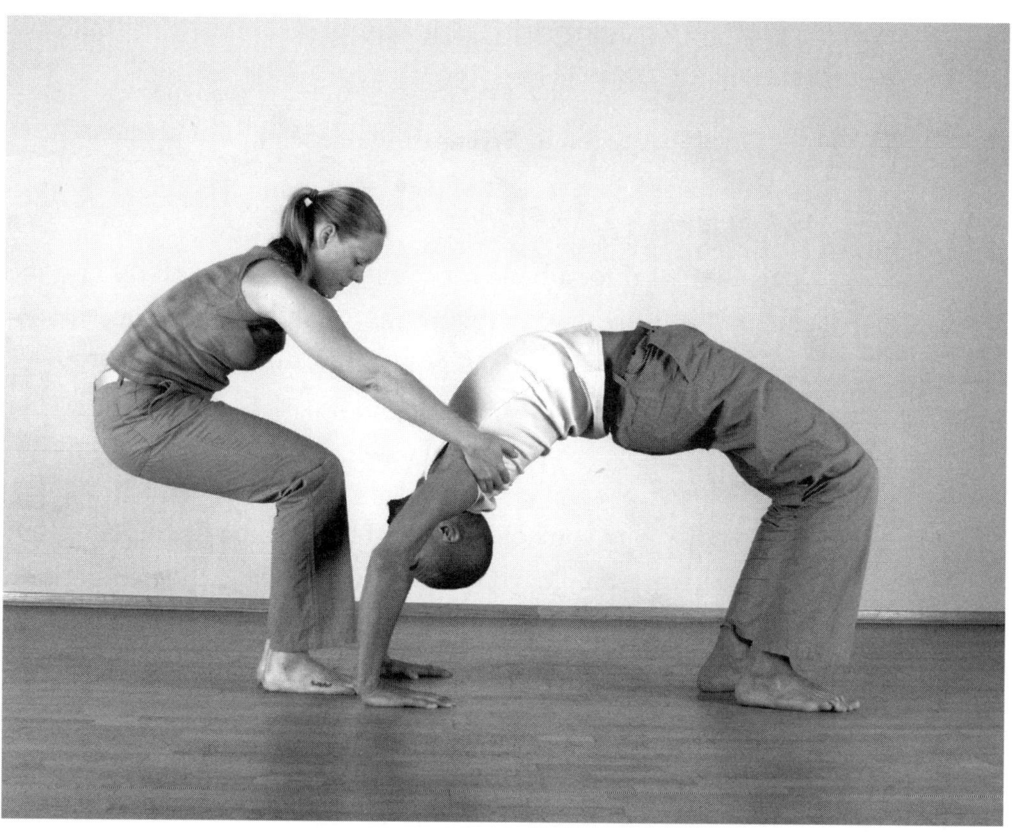

17. Advanced Back Bridge (with leg raised)

Flexibility-stretch. Strength. Balance.

Movement

Begin this as if for a basic back bridge and then push up into the full bridge. Raise one leg toward the ceiling and hold the position. Lower the leg again and get stable, then raise the other leg. This can be done with your supporting foot flat, or on your toes.

Breathing

Gauge how long you hold the raised-leg position by counting your breaths. For example, you might try holding each leg high for a count of 5 full cycles of inhalation and exhalation.

Pointers

Keep driving your hips upward as you raise your leg, as if you are pushing the ball of your extended foot toward the ceiling.

Health and Fitness Benefits

As well as the benefits already described for bridges, this movement will strengthen you for many capoeira techniques, such as walkovers, "macacos," "S dobrados," and various types of "moenda" for which a strong, flexible spine and shoulders are a great help.

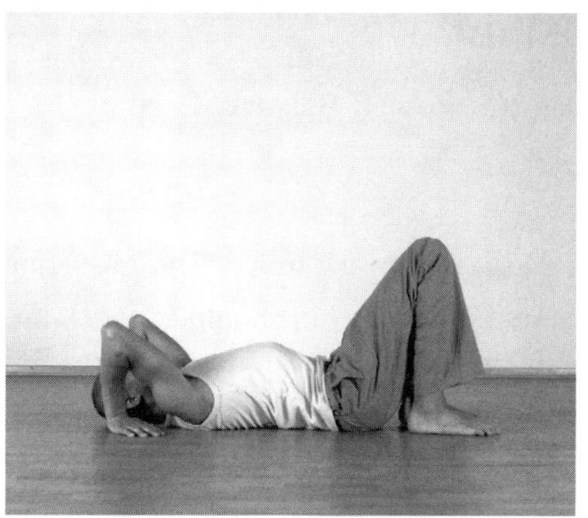
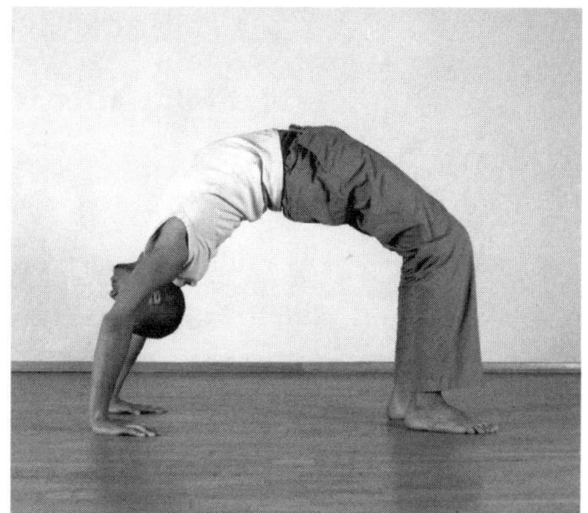
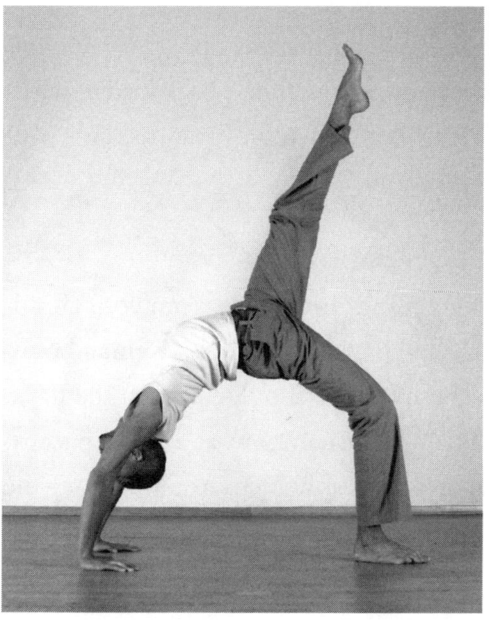
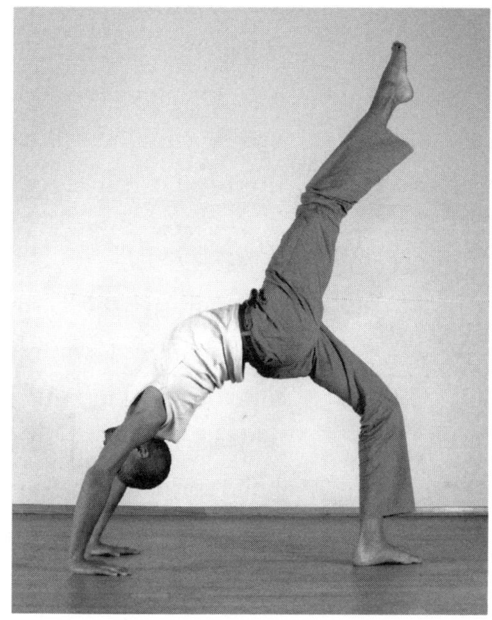

18. Back Bridge Push-Ups

Flexibility-stretch. Strength. Power. Balance. Cardio.

Movement

Do a full basic back bridge. At the end of the movement, take your chin to your chest and lower yourself until your shoulders touch the floor, then drop your hips and lower your back flat on the floor. Immediately raise your hips and push straight back up again to a full bridge with arms locked out straight. Repeat 10, 20, or 30 times.

Breathing

Inhale on the way down, and exhale on the way up. Try to get into a groove, inhaling and exhaling in time with the back bridge push-ups. If you find full nasal breathing difficult, inhale through your nose and exhale through your mouth.

Pointers

You can vary this by pressing up and down only from your shoulders, without lowering your back between each rep. Remember to dip your chin in onto your chest so your shoulders reach the floor. This variation is a bridge push-up you can do at a rapid pace to build springiness and power into your shoulders. You might try the regular back bridge push-ups more slowly, concentrating on your breathing and squeezing out the movement at the top of the bridge.

Health and Fitness Benefits

Back bridge push-ups build power and flexibility in your back, shoulders, wrists, and thighs. This is a whole-body exercise that uses all your major muscle groups and is highly recommended as a capoeira conditioning exercise.

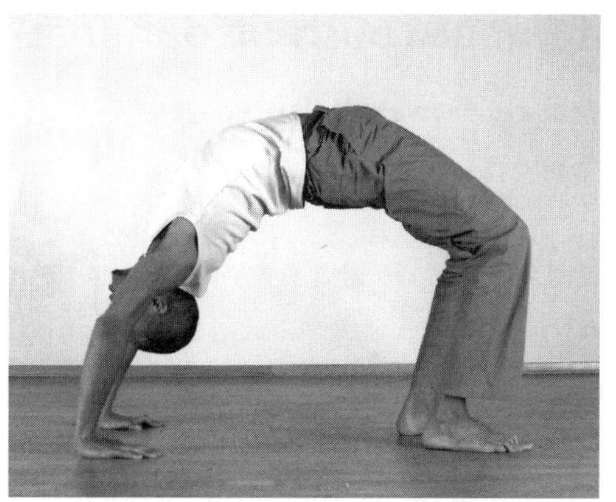

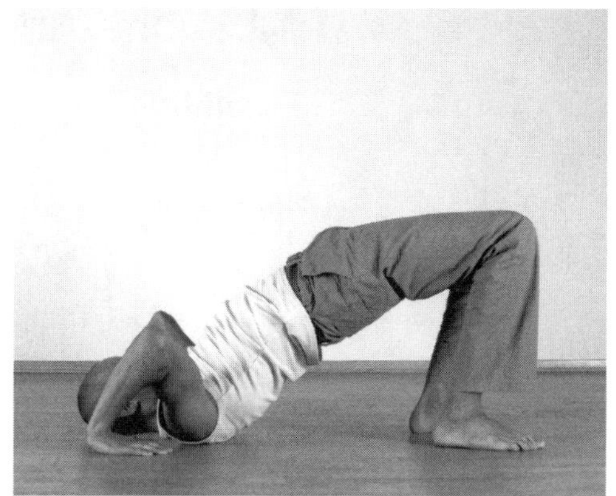

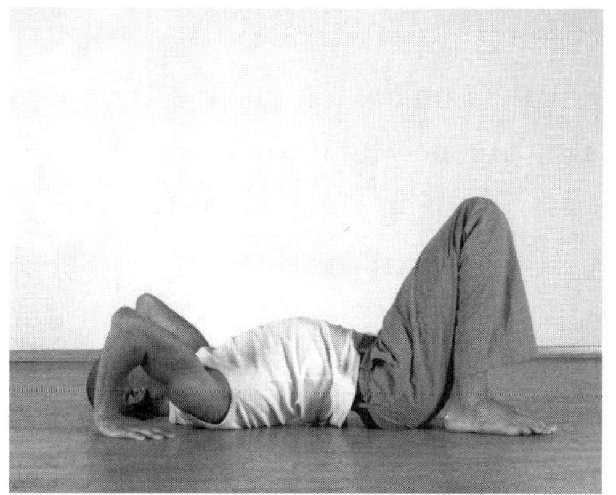

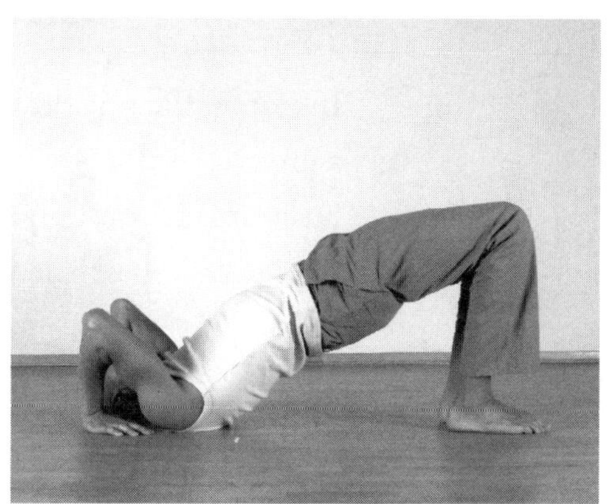

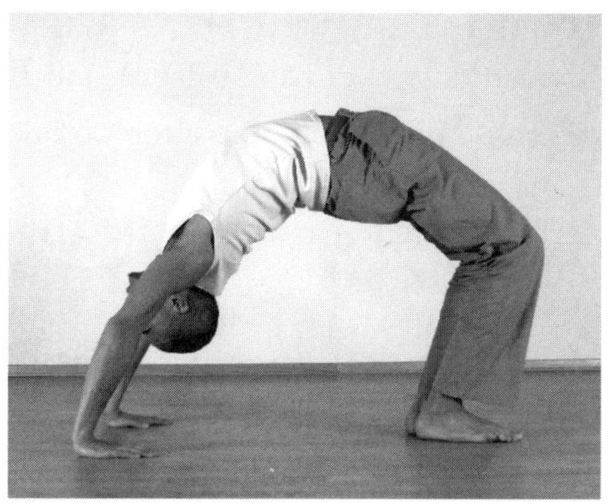

19. One-Armed Bridge (push-up optional)

Flexibility-stretch. Strength. Power. Balance.

Movement

From a full bridge position raise one arm and lay it on your chest. Replace it and change arm to the other side. If you feel inspired, try lowering for a one-armed bridge push-up. This is an advanced movement and will be interesting as a variation only to those who are very confident in the other exercises of the bridge sequence.

Breathing

Inhale on the way down, and exhale on the way up. Try to get into a groove, inhaling and exhaling in time with the one-armed bridge push-ups. If you find full nasal breathing difficult, inhale through your nose and exhale through your mouth.

Pointers

Use your fingertips to maintain your balance, and keep the fingers spread as wide as possible to help with this.

Health and Fitness Benefits

As a static movement this is great for strength and balance, and as a push-up it intensifies the exercise by isolating the effort to one arm and shoulder.

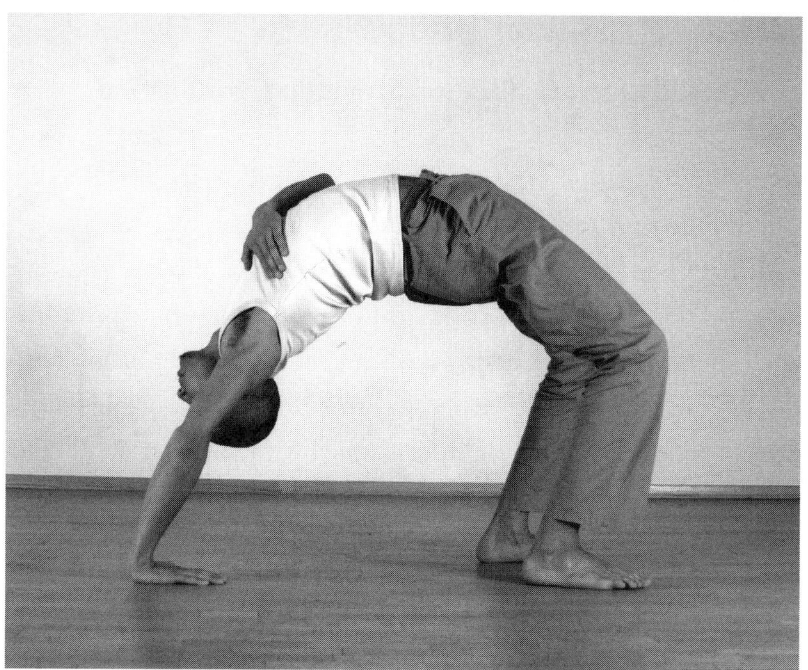

20. No Cheat Bridge

Flexibility-stretch. Balance. Strength. Coordination.

Movement

This is called a no cheat bridge because in capoeira you don't touch your back to the ground. Start in cocorinha, and place your left hand on the floor behind your left foot. Raise your hips as high as you can and reach back over your head with your right hand, looking behind yourself between your arms. Keeping your hips high, place the right hand on the floor parallel with your left hand. The fingertips of your two hands should be pointed toward each other. Now rest the weight on your right hand, bring up the left hand, drop your hips, and move into a cocorinha. Repeat the same sequence back in the other direction.

Breathing

Breathe freely.

Pointers

Always do the wrist warm-up (No. 8–11) before doing this movement and preferably the ginga with a reverse twist (No. 5) to warm up your waist and shoulders. This is an exercise best done while you are fully warmed up. Note that by aiming the fingertips of the two hands toward each other you will avoid twisting your wrists. If you find it very difficult, simply get to the stage where you reach back, hold that position, taking 5 deep breaths, and then drop your hips and go into cocorinha again, repeating this on the other side. As your body adapts, you can move on to the full movement.

Health and Fitness Benefits

The front of your body gets a very effective stretch while your spine is arched. Mobility in your shoulders will be increased, which will enhance the fluidity of your movements. Your wrist and ankle strength increases. The movement has overall benefits for your circulation, and many glands and internal organs.

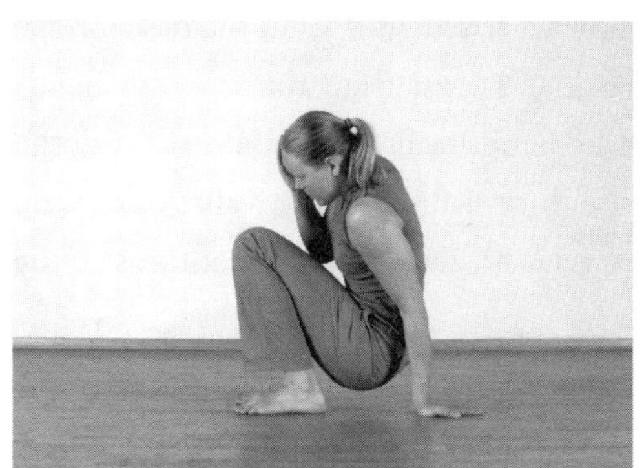

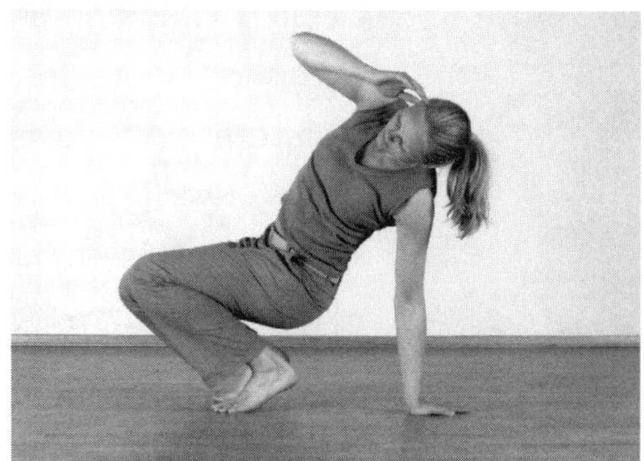

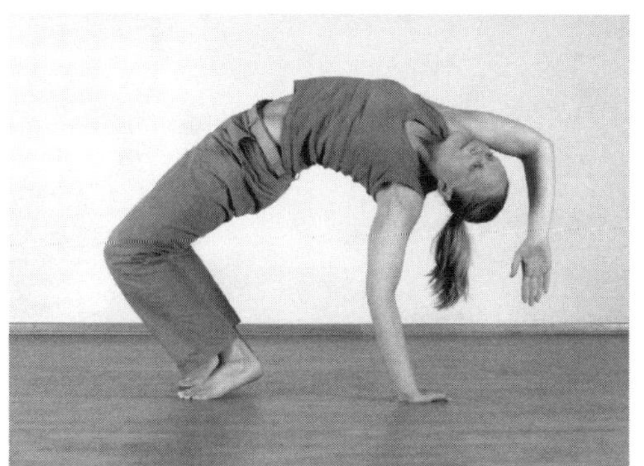

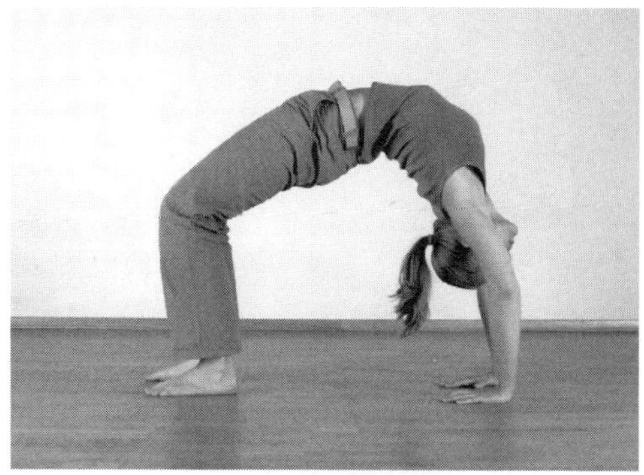

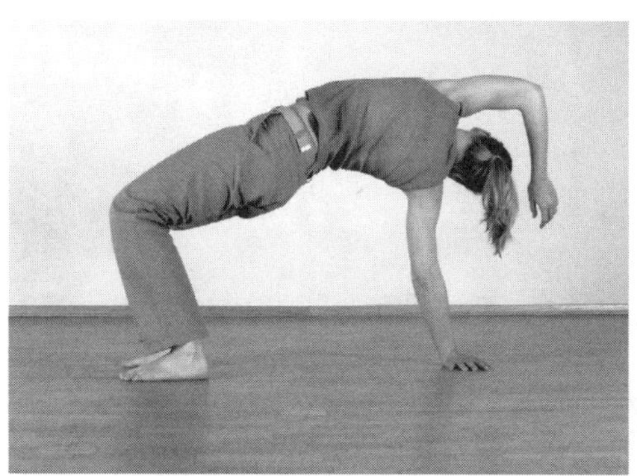

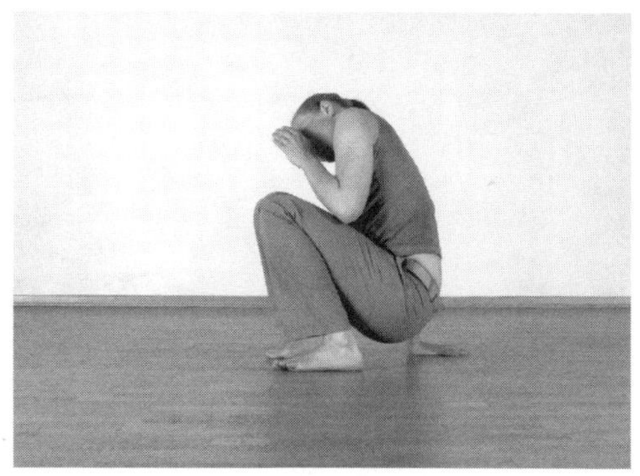

21. Wall Wheel Bridge

Flexibility-stretch. Strength. Balance.

Movement

Get into a position with your back to the wall, as in the basic bridge warm-up (No. 12). Lean back and press the palms of your hands against the wall, then hand by hand, walk yourself down until the crown of your head is on the floor. Immediately walk yourself up again until you are standing relaxed. Do 5 or 10 repetitions of the wall wheel bridge.

Breathing

Breathe freely.

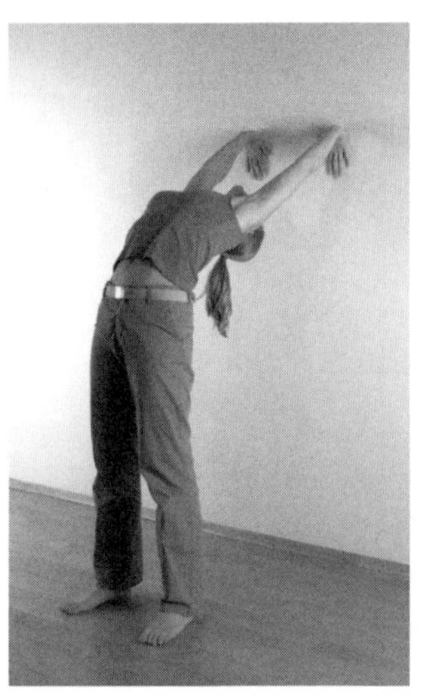
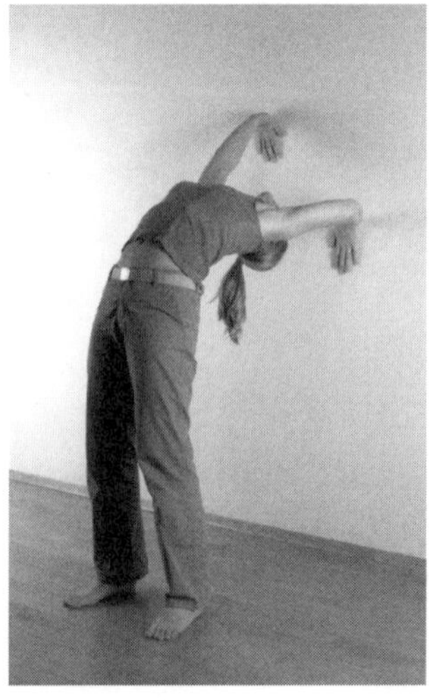
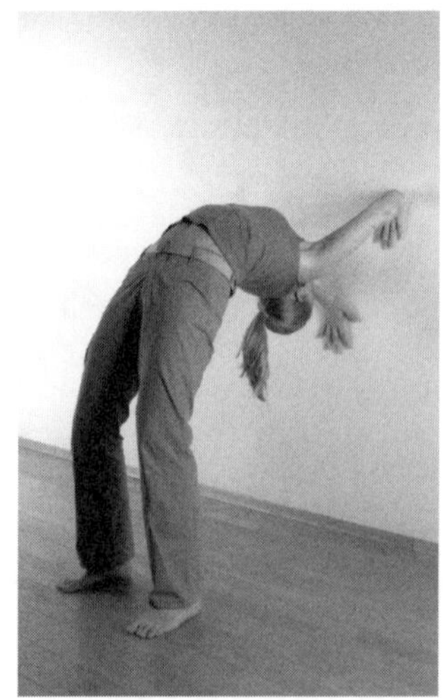

Pointers

Safety is an issue here as you do not want to slip down the wall and bang your head on the floor. Make sure you are a good distance from the wall, not too far, not too close. Lead with your hands so that they get to the floor before your head does. Don't stand on a rug that moves or do this against a door that someone might open. If your hands are slippery, moisten them slightly so they don't slip on the wall.

Health and Fitness Benefits

This is another whole-body exercise that conditions everything from your gluteus maximus to your abs. If you combine this with the basic forward bend (No. 13), it is a very good all-around strengthener, stretch, and toner for your legs, back, and shoulders. It also expands your chest and forces your body to work in movement through the bridge position.

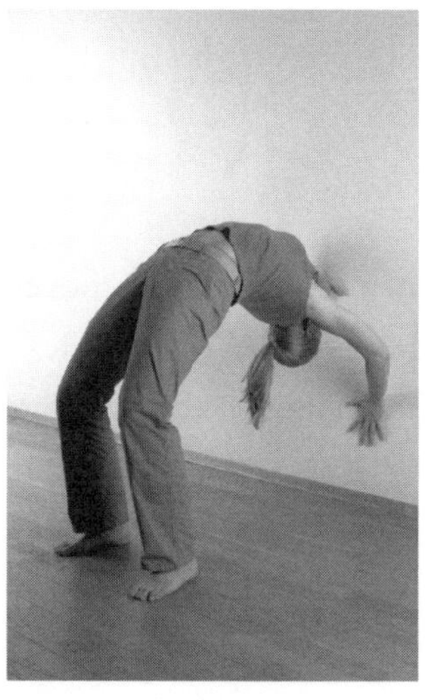
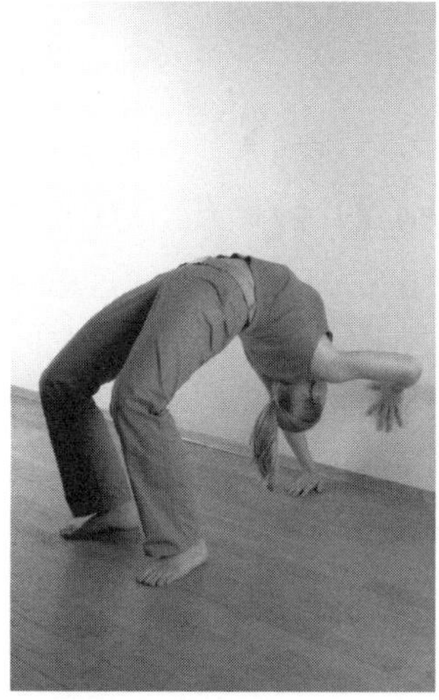
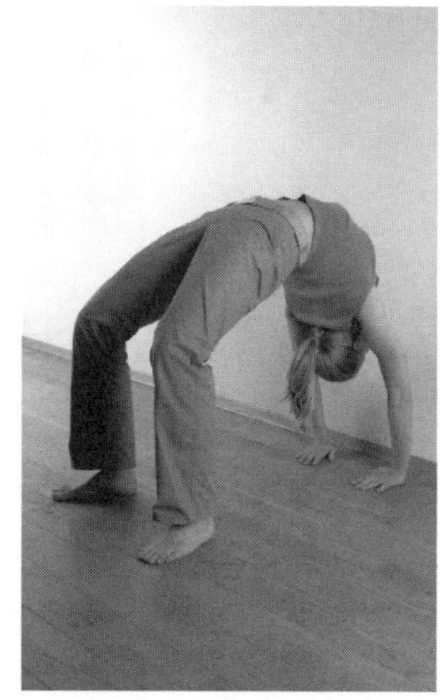

22. Bridge Walking

Flexibility-stretch. Strength. Balance. Cardio. Coordination.

Movement

Do the basic back bridge and then walk forward one hand and one foot at a time. If you are in an enclosed space, walk forward a few steps and then walk backward a few steps. Try to continue bridge walking for 2 or 3 minutes, after which time you will probably be exhausted, and you can lie flat on your back and squeeze your knees up to your chest.

Breathing

Breathe freely.

Pointers

For most people this is a tough exercise, so work slowly but surely. Try to breathe and focus and enjoy each step, thinking how much more lithe and flexible it is making you, rather than yearning for it to be over. In this way you gain maximum benefit from the movement and it's more fun. Keep your neck relaxed with your head hanging down between your arms.

Health and Fitness Benefits

The benefits here are the same as for a basic back bridge; the movement will increase coordination skills and build strength and flexibility in your back, shoulders, wrists, legs, and hips. Bridge walking is an excellent exercise for capoeira.

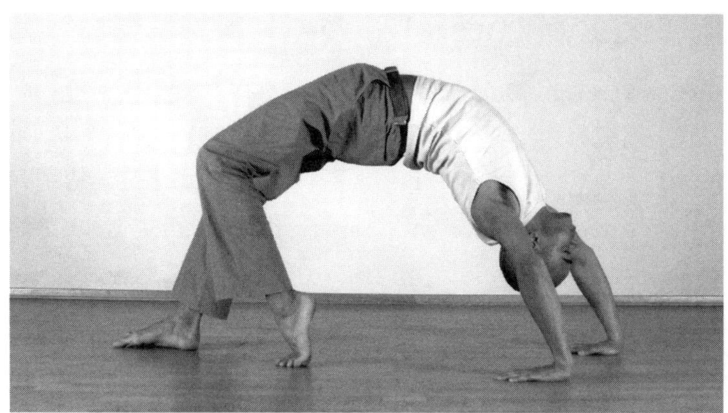

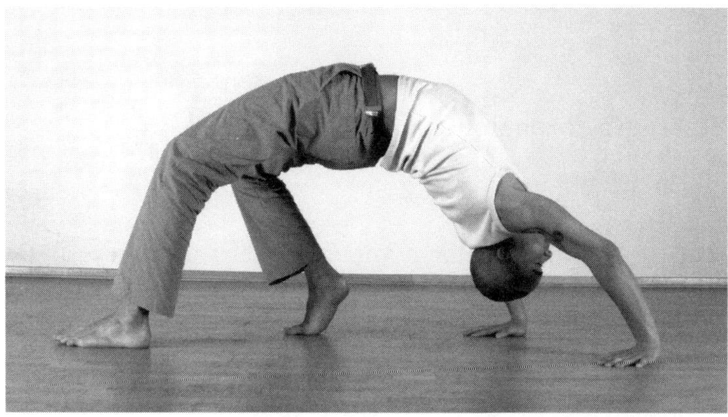

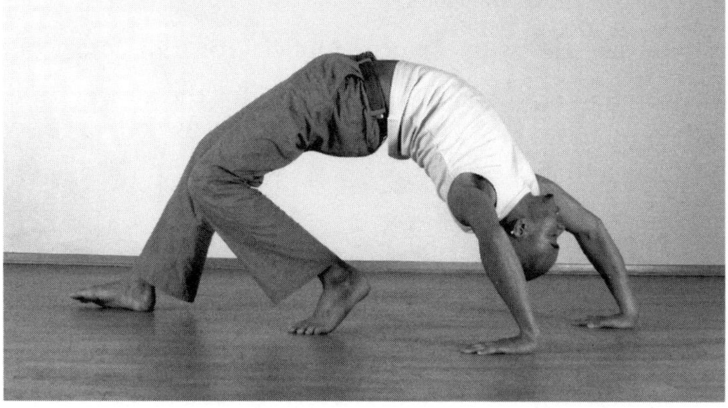

23. Esquiva Lateral

Flexibility-stretch. Balance.

Movement

Stand with your feet shoulder-width apart, feet parallel. Bend one knee and support your weight on the palm of your hand on the same side as your bent knee. For a full stretch you can extend your other arm out straight beyond your head. Keep your hips low and hold the position for 6 breaths. Change and do the same thing to the other side.

Breathing

Take deep breaths through the nose.

Pointers

The foot of the bent leg can be pointed outward slightly in alignment with the leg. The other leg should be completely straight and the hips low. Don't let your upper shoulder slouch forward, and try to keep your whole body in alignment.

Health and Fitness Benefits

A good lateral stretch for the spine, beneficial for toning up your spinal nerves. This exercise is also a warm-up for the aú workout.

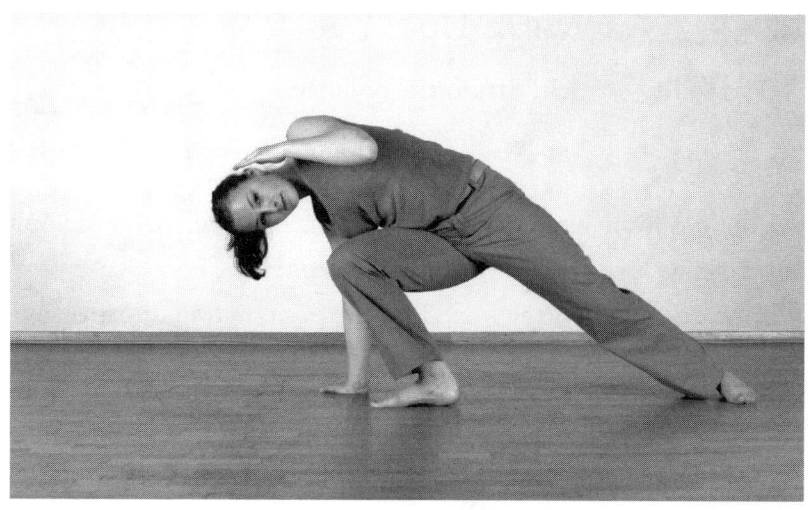

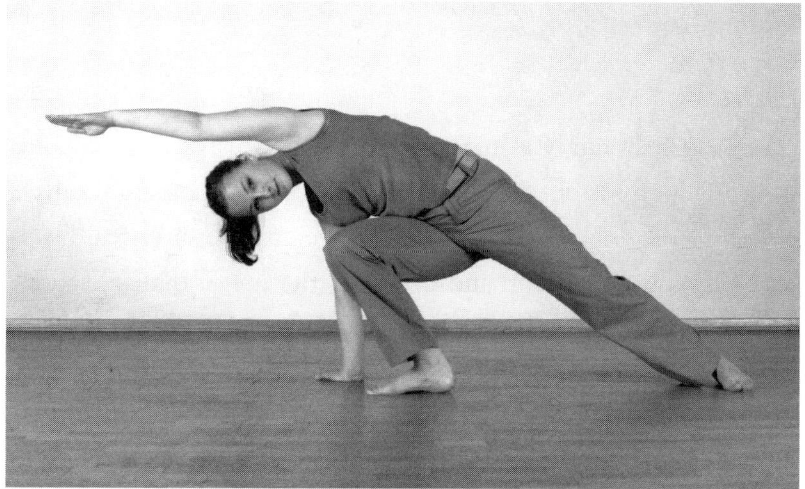

24. Aú Warm-Up

Flexibility-stretch. Strength. Balance.

Movement

Do the esquiva lateral (No. 23) position. Place the palm of your outstretched arm beyond your head and onto the floor. Raise your straight leg and point the toe. Hold the position for 6 breaths, and then drop back into the esquiva lateral position. You can do the whole sequence six times, three to the left and three to the right.

Breathing

Do deep nasal breathing, concentrating on staying relaxed while holding your balance.

Pointers

Your weight should be equally distributed between your two hands and your support foot. Keep the upper foot's toe pointed to give a stretch to the ankle. To give an extra stretch to your calf and support leg, you can rise up and down on the toe of that foot a few times if you like. Your support leg will straighten in this movement, and then revert to its bent position when you drop into esquiva lateral again.

Health and Fitness Benefits

This movement gives a lateral stretch to the spine, and strengthens your wrists and shoulders. The rising and lowering stretch will give your calves and ankles a workout. This is also an excellent movement for your balance.

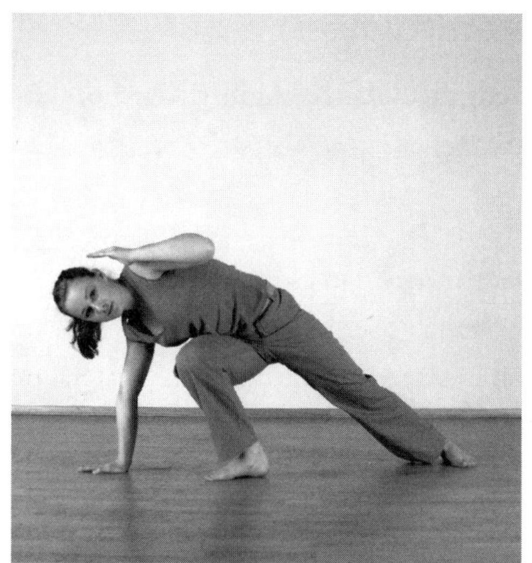

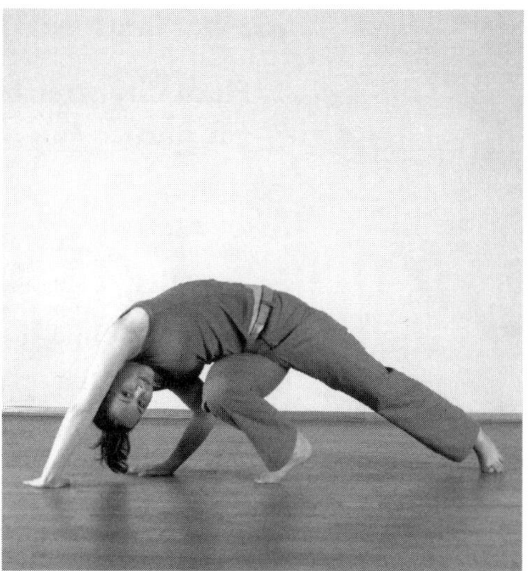

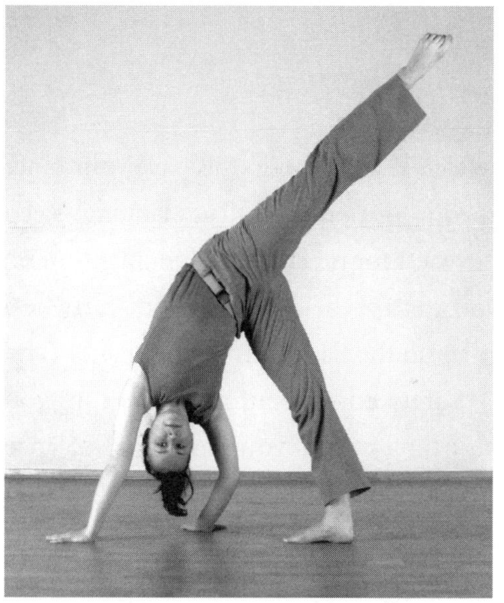

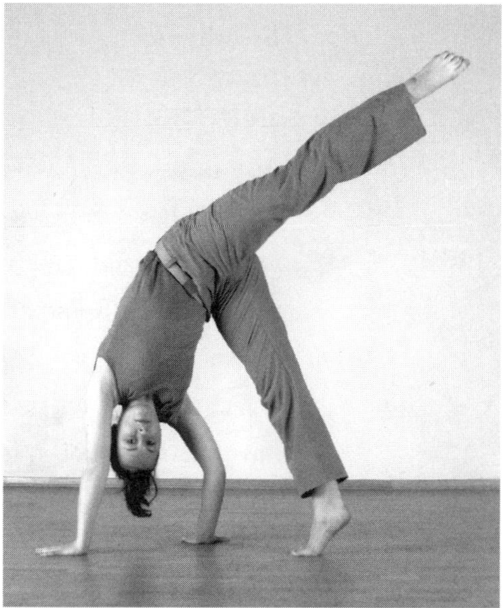

25. Aú Normal (cartwheel)

Flexibility-stretch. Strength. Balance. Agility. Cardio. Fat Burner. Coordination.

Movement

Stand with feet shoulder-width apart. Do esquiva lateral (No. 23), then aú warm-up (No. 24), launch over in a cartwheel so you end up in an aú stretch on the other side, drop into an esquiva lateral on that side, and come up into a standing position. Do the same thing back in the other direction. Repeat 10, 20, or 30 times. Always aú in both directions to develop balance in your musculature.

Breathing

Breathe freely.

Pointers

As you see, the aú is a cartwheel. When you do this have your inner support hand quite close to your foot on takeoff and landing. Keep your legs straight and use the waist for precision and momentum on the way over. Remember, you control the cartwheel—the cartwheel doesn't control you. Always aú on the flat palms of your hands (and warm up your wrists first). Safety consideration: Make sure you have plenty of room for this exercise, so if you tumble off balance you don't hit anything.

You can vary this by doing an aú normal, but keep the palms of your hands on the floor and simply aú from side to side, working your waist with the body always aligned (the hands remain on the ground as you flip from side to side, 10 to 20 repetitions). This variation is a great aerobic exercise and will build strength in your arms and flexibility in your spine and hips.

Health and Fitness Benefits

A good exercise for your oblique muscles. Great for balance and coordination. Doing this with many repetitions will build strength in your arms and shoulders and help build stamina. Aú is an important movement in capoeira.

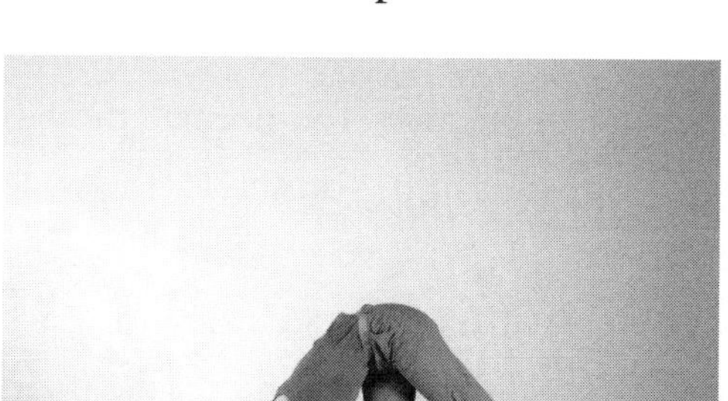

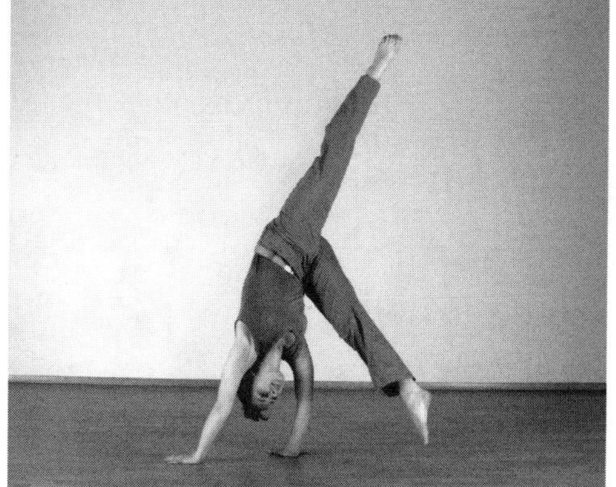

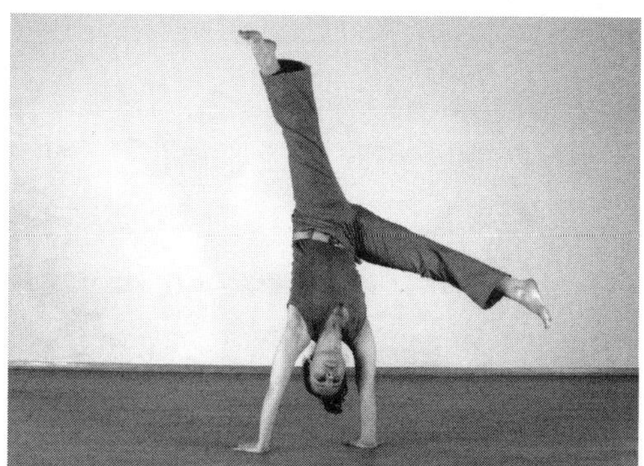

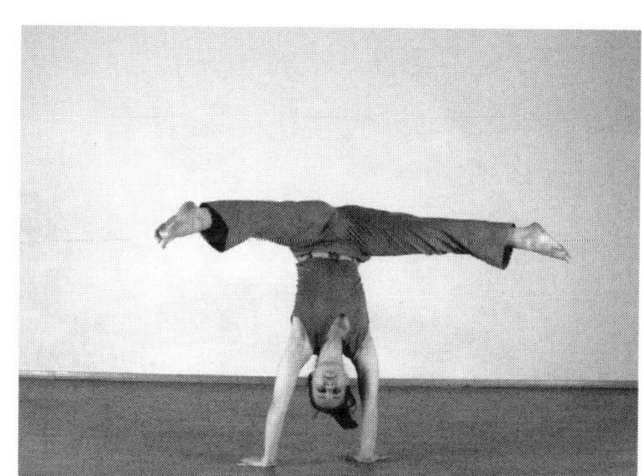

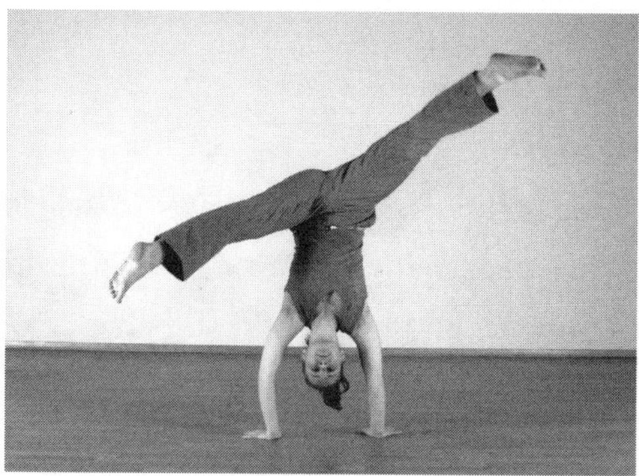

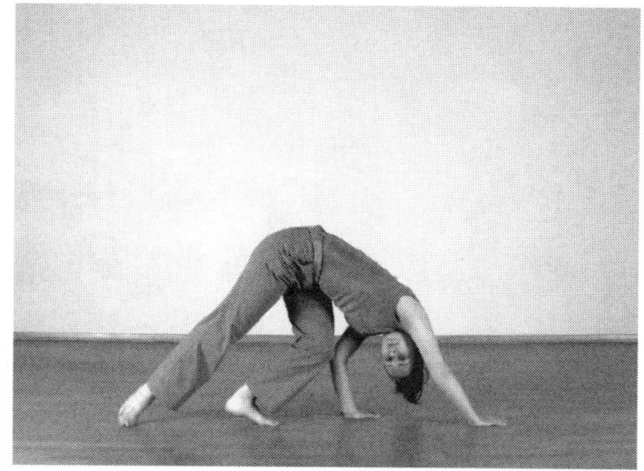

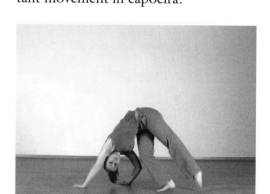

26. Aú Walkback

Flexibility-stretch. Strength. Balance. Agility. Cardio. Fat Burner. Coordination.

Movement

This movement is exactly the same in practice as aú normal, though because you step back for the initial pushoff, you stay in the same spot as you do the movement.

Stand with your feet shoulder-width apart. Step one leg back behind the other and place the flat palm of your hand on the floor. Lift your front leg and push off from the back leg into an aú. If you push off from your left leg you will land on the right and vice versa.

Breathing

Breathe freely.

Pointers

This is an exercise you can do in a small space (because you stay in the same spot). Land as lightly as you can. Once you have learned to land lightly and stay in the same spot, you can even do it in a small hotel room. Use your waist as much as you can and learn to flip your body from side to side keeping the hands close to the feet and doing most of the work with the waist.

Health and Fitness Benefits

This is a good exercise for your oblique muscles. Great for balance and coordination. Doing this with many repetitions will build strength in your arms and shoulders and help build stamina.

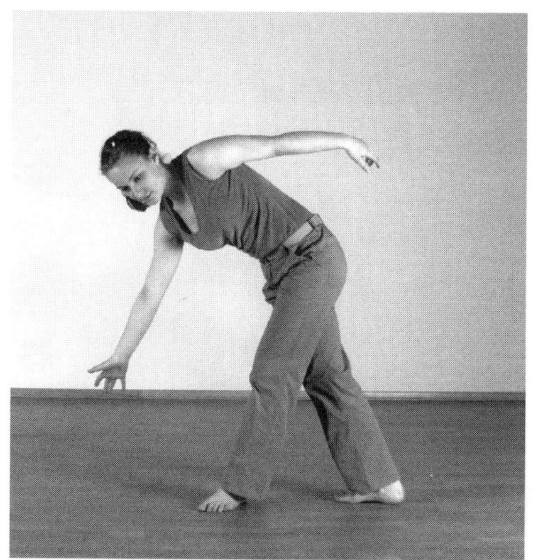

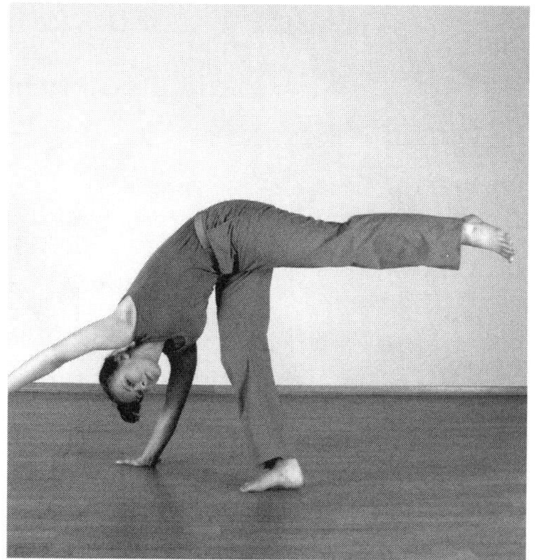

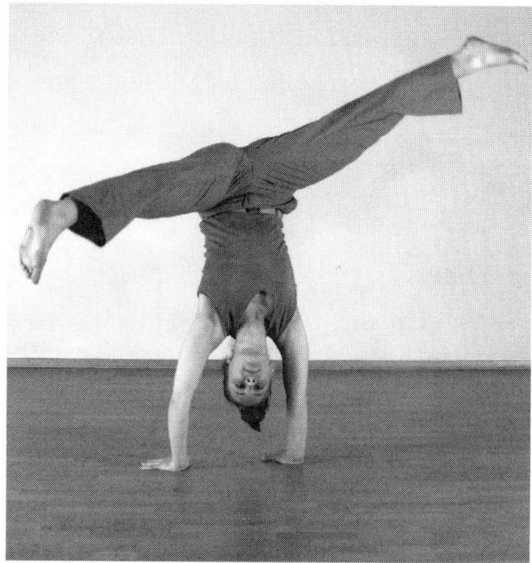

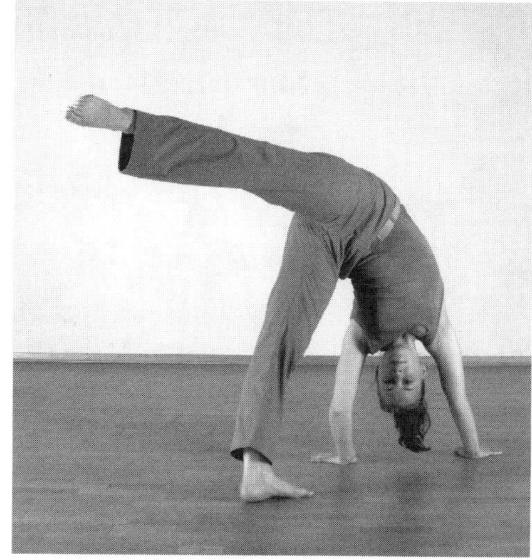

27. Aú Push-Ups

Flexibility-stretch. Strength. Balance. Cardio.

Movement

Start off in aú warm-up (No. 24) position. Bend both your arms and touch the top of your head on the floor, then push back up into the straight-armed aú warm-up position. Repeat 10 times to the right and 10 times to the left.

Breathing

Inhale on the way down, and exhale as you push back up.

Pointers

Have your hands firmly planted on their palms. Try to lock both arms out straight when you reach the top of the movement. Keep your whole body in alignment. Go up and down slowly and steadily, in unison with your breathing.

Health and Fitness Benefits

This builds strength in the shoulders and triceps. It is also a good strength builder for the back, and as preparation for the bananeira push-up.

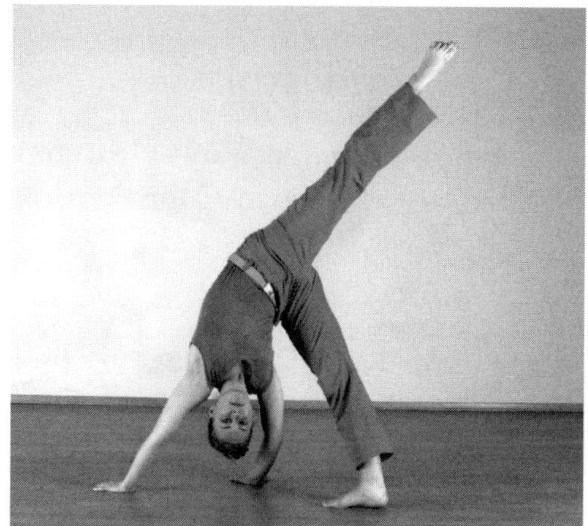

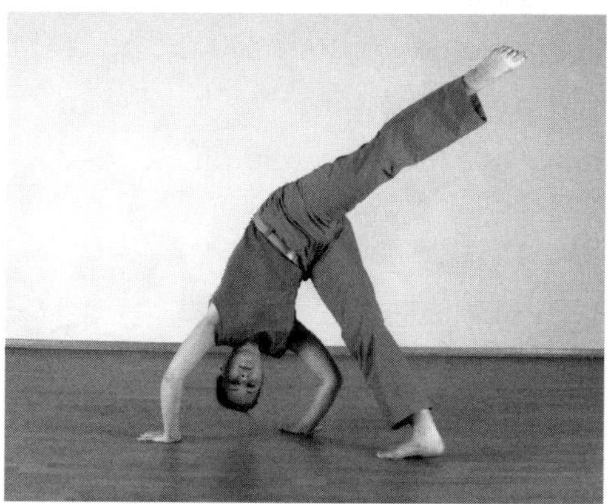

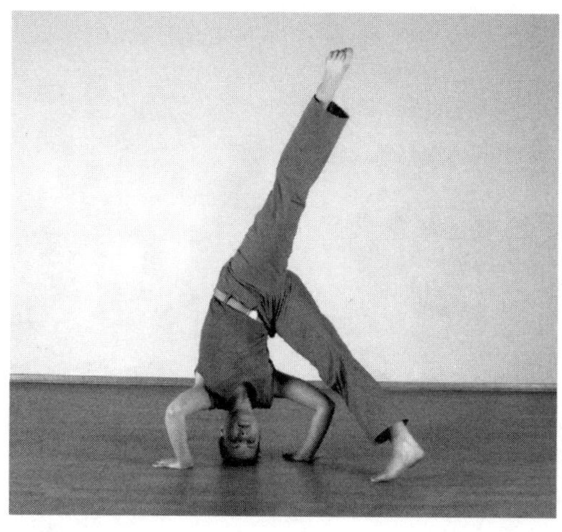

28. Aú Pistols

Flexibility-stretch. Power. Strength. Balance. Cardio. Fat Burner. Coordination.

Movement

Do aú normal (No. 25), launching off from your right foot, landing on your left foot. When you land on your left foot, keep the right leg extended out directly in front of you. Drop into a one-legged squat and push up again. Without putting your right leg on the ground, launch into an aú normal in the other direction, landing on your right foot. Do the squat (pistol) with left leg extended and come up again, then back in the other direction. Repeat the movement 10, 20, or 30 times.

Breathing

Breathe freely.

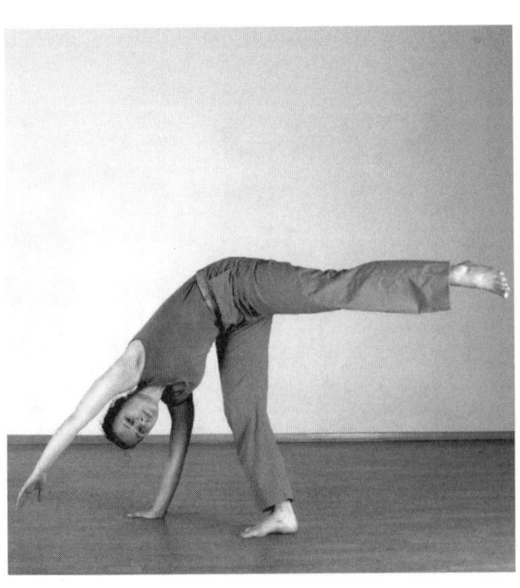

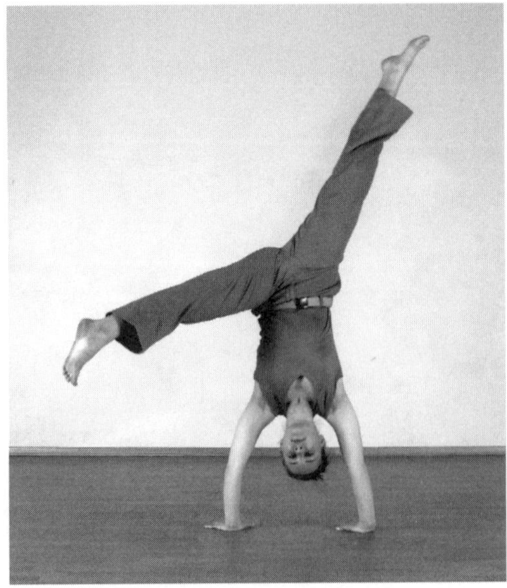

Pointers

You can up the intensity of this sequence by increasing the repetition of pistols between aú normals. For example, do five pistol squats between aús instead of one. Keep your extended leg directly out straight in front of you, and you can bring your hands forward for balance. Keep your supporting foot flat to maximize balance and the stretch for your ankle.

Health and Fitness Benefits

In this exercise you combine all the benefits derived from the aú normal with the incredible power-building potential of the one-legged (pistol) squat. It is an excellent exercise for overall balance and forces you to focus on landing from your aú normal with enough control to remain standing on one leg. High repetitions of pistols will build springiness in your legs and power for kicking and is beneficial to your stamina.

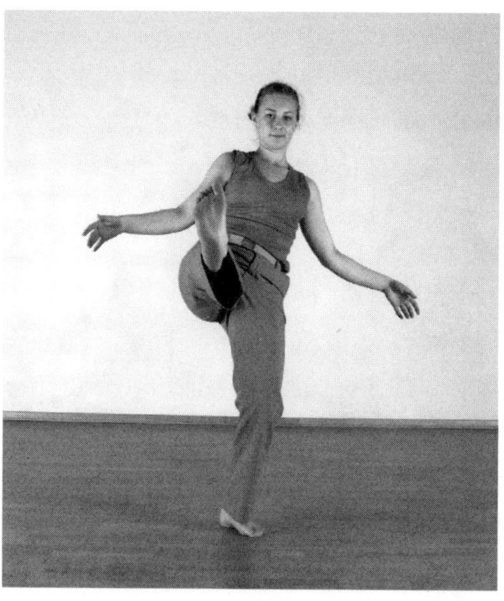

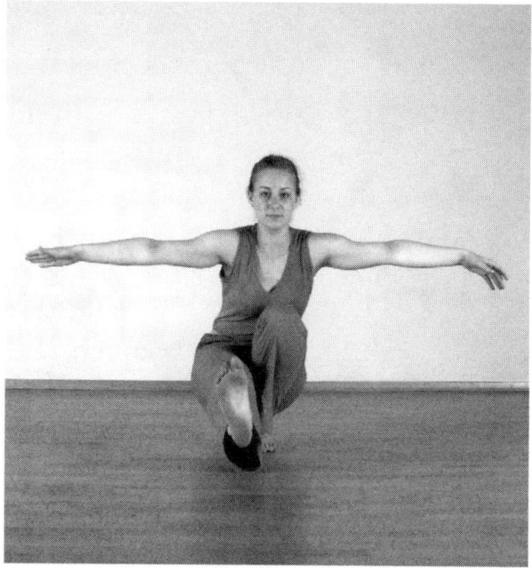

29. Negativa Lateral

Flexibility-stretch. Strength. Balance.

Movement

Do an esquiva lateral position. Stretch one arm out beyond your head and place the palm of the hand on the floor. Turn the knee of your bent leg inward and drop down low so that you are virtually parallel with the floor. You are looking to the front with your head poised in the middle of your arms. Come up into cocorinha and do the same thing to the other side. Repeat the process 10 times.

Breathing

Inhale as you move into the position, and exhale as you move back up into the cocorinha. It is also advisable to hold the position for two or three inhalations and exhalations, to get a static workout for strength, a good stretch, and endurance.

Pointers

Don't lie on the ground here. Your hip and lower leg shouldn't be touching the floor, but poised just above it. Get into a groove and switch from side to side more rapidly for a good strength-building workout that will increase aerobic capacity.

Health and Fitness Benefits

This will build power and springiness in your arms, and flexibility in your shoulders. Like esquiva lateral, negativa lateral stretches your spine laterally, which is very beneficial to the spinal nerves. The cocorinha between negativa movements is also good for your lower spine and sacroiliac joints.

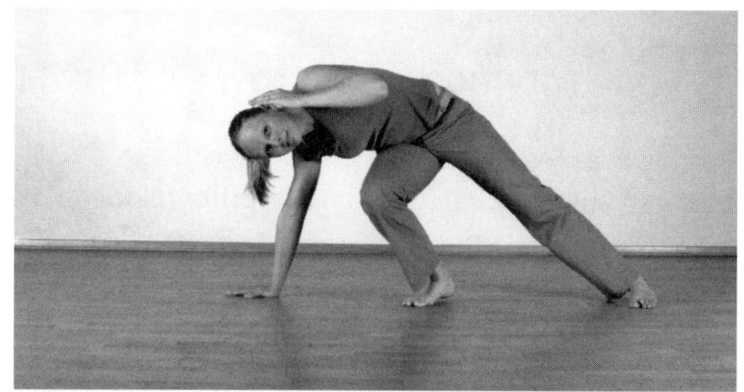

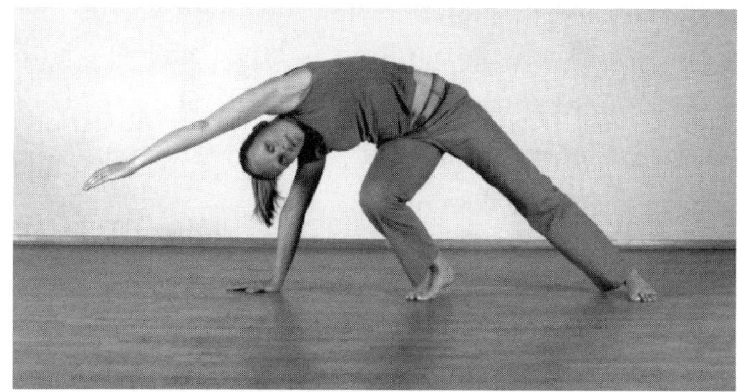

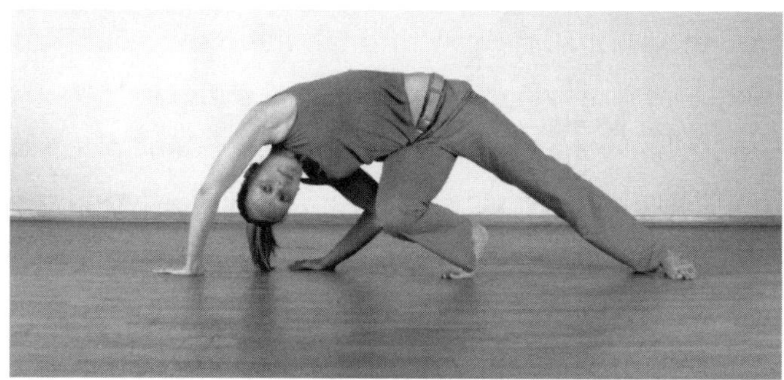

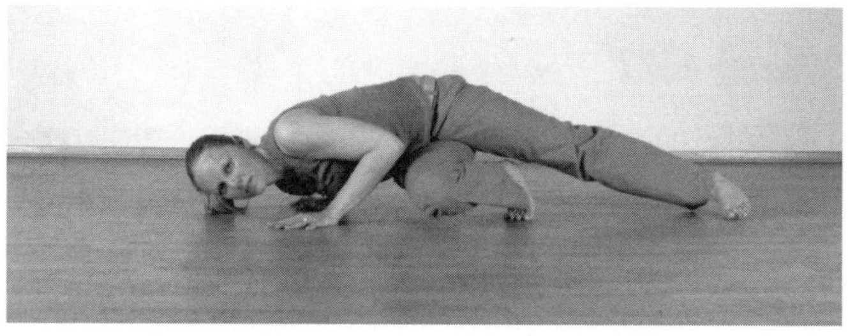

30. Moenda with Crown of the Head on the Floor

Flexibility-stretch. Strength. Agility. Coordination.

Movement

Cocorinha (No. 1), then do a negativa lateral (No. 29) and place the crown of your head on the floor between your hands. Arching your back a little, walk your feet and trunk around behind you in a semi-circle (keeping your head and the palms of your hands on the ground) until you are in a negativa lateral on the other side, then push up into a cocorinha (No. 1) again. Do exactly the same thing back in the other direction.

Breathing

Breathe deeply and freely.

Pointers

Face the front all the way through this movement. It is your whole body that is moving 180 degrees in a semi-circle back behind your head, while your head stays in exactly the same place, between your hands, facing in the same direction. Work slowly and steadily, breathing for concentration. If you reach a sticking point, try not to collapse and give up, but relax and analyze the situation, thinking what you have to do with your feet, hips, and waist to get your trunk around to the other side.

Health and Fitness Benefits

This unusual movement is nowhere near as difficult as it looks. It frees up the hips, spine, neck, and shoulders, and works the body through an unusual range of movement. Mobility will be increased, as will muscular strength.

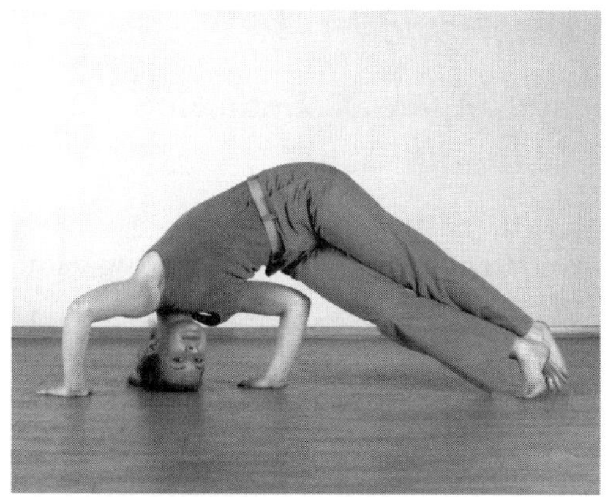
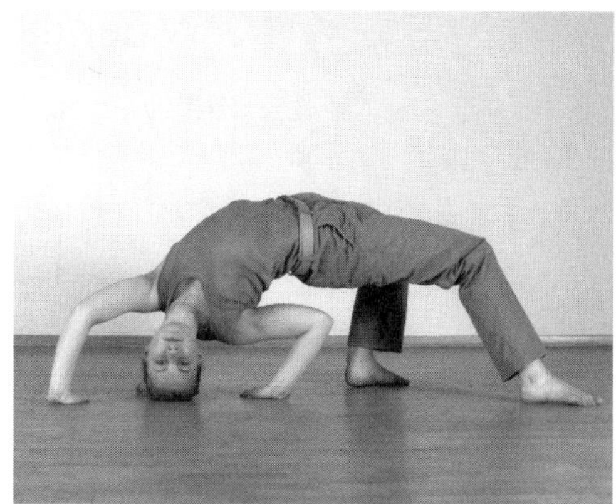
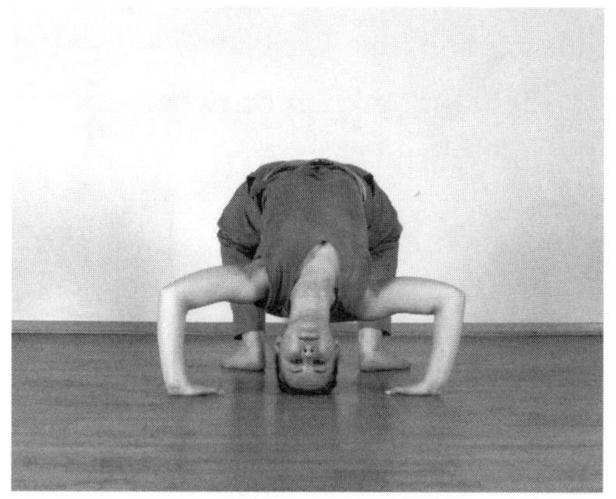
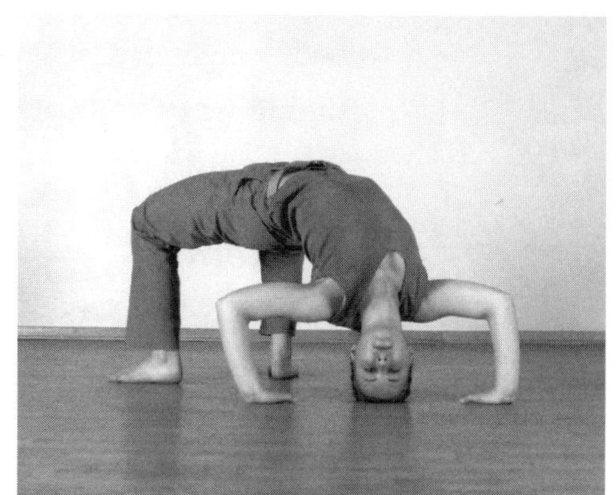
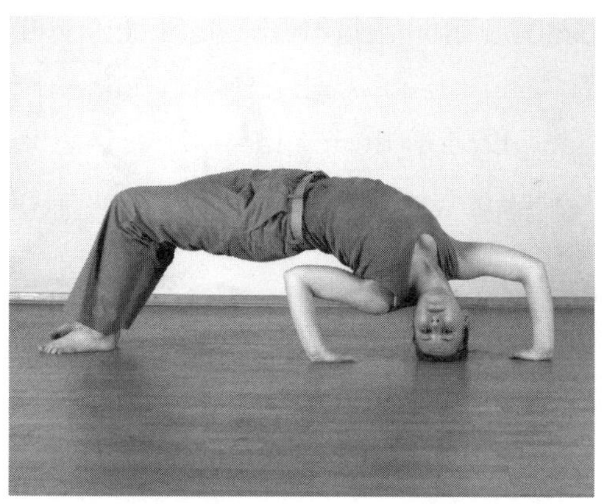
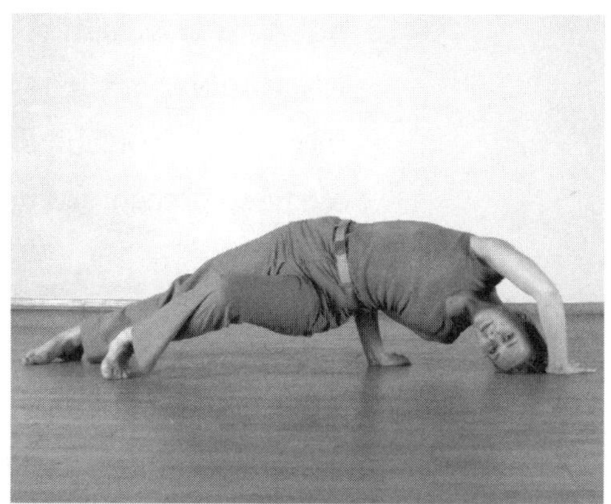

31. Moenda on the Hands

Flexibility-stretch. Strength. Agility. Coordination.

Movement

This movement, like negativa lateral, is perfect for the low game of capoeira (jogo de baixo). You begin the movement in the same way as No. 30, but this time do not place the crown of your head on the floor. Instead, bring your chin in to your chest, so that your body weight is distributed between your hands and feet. Walk your feet around in a semi-circle behind yourself while maintaining your body weight evenly between hands and feet. The back of your head should be poised parallel to the floor, an inch or two above the floor, all the way through the movement.

Breathing

As for No. 30.

Pointers

The same as for No. 30, and the angle of your head will remain so you can look in front of you in between your arms and hands. Do not rest the back of your head and shoulders on the floor, although it's possible they may brush against the floor lightly as you do the movement. Your hips remain quite low during moenda; it is a different movement from the bridge (where the hips are thrust higher).

Health and Fitness Benefits

These are the same as for No. 30, with the added work that your wrists are doing. The movement is increasing the range of motion in your shoulders, is rotating the spine, and is an excellent toning exercise for the whole upper body. Moenda can be hard work but is highly recommended for capoeira conditioning.

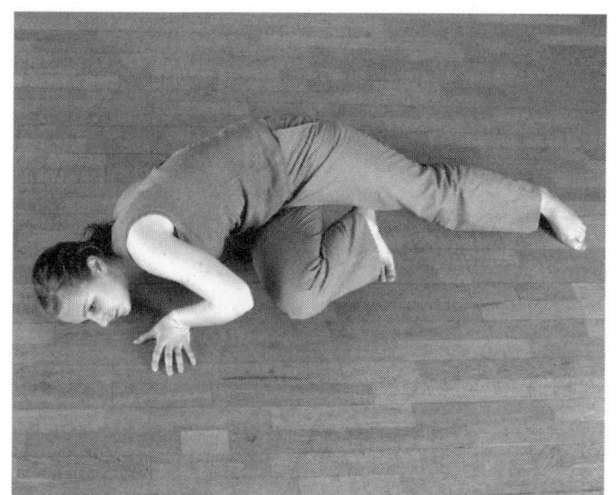

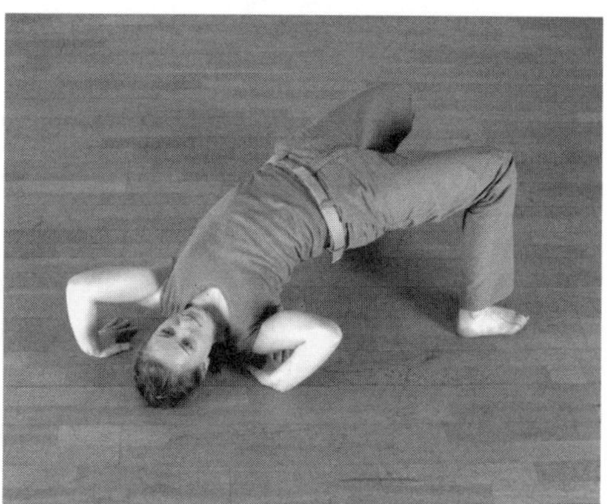

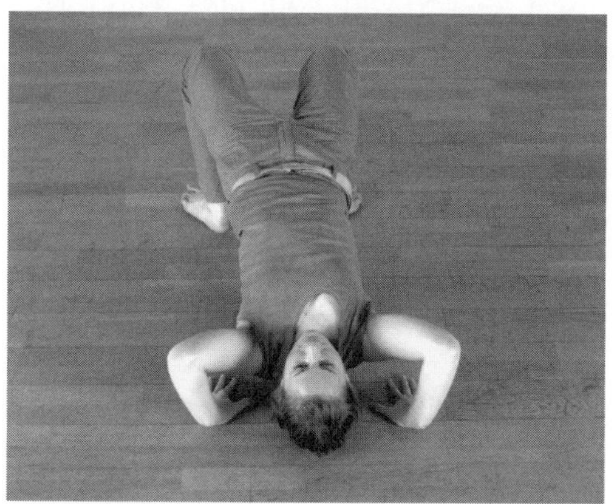

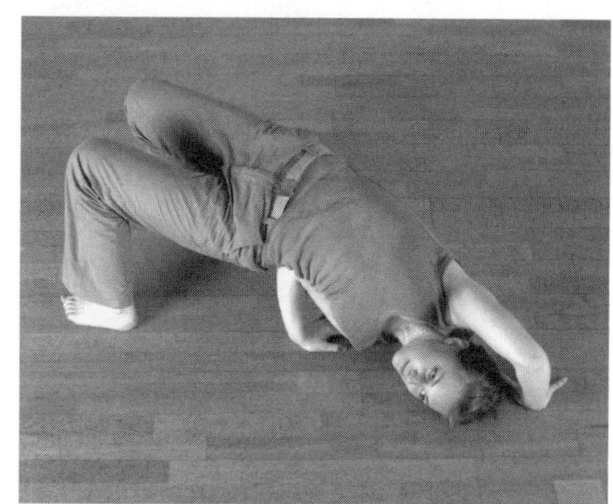

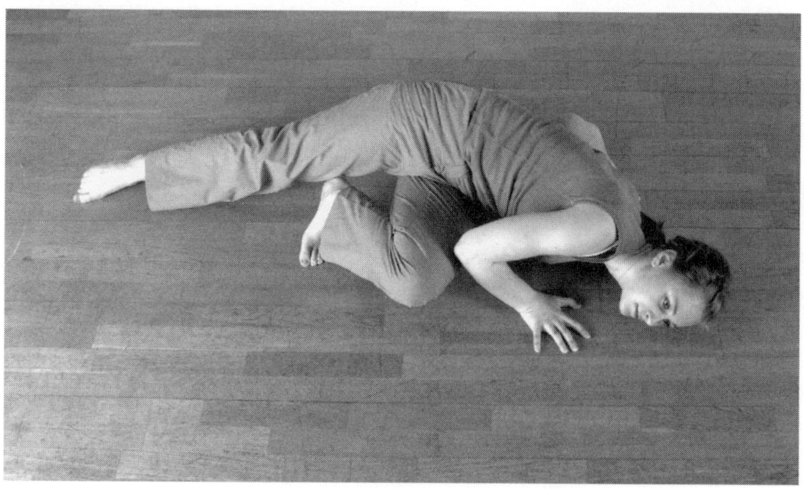

32. Queda de Quatro-Chapa

Flexibility-stretch.

Movement

This is a front kick delivered from the floor. Do a cocorinha (No. 1). Keeping your feet flat on the floor, tip back onto your hands, with your fingertips directed away from your body. Your body weight is now evenly distributed between your two hands and two feet, hence the name "queda de quatro" (falling on four). Immediately raise one leg and thrust it upward with your hips. This thrust upward of your straight leg is the kick called "chapa." Collapse your hips back down into queda de quatro again and thrust up your straight leg kick on the other side. This can be done from a flat foot or on the toes, as demonstrated in the photo. Repeat side to side steadily.

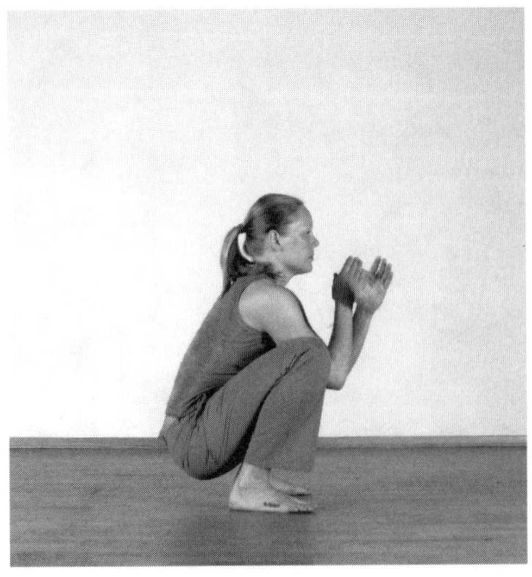

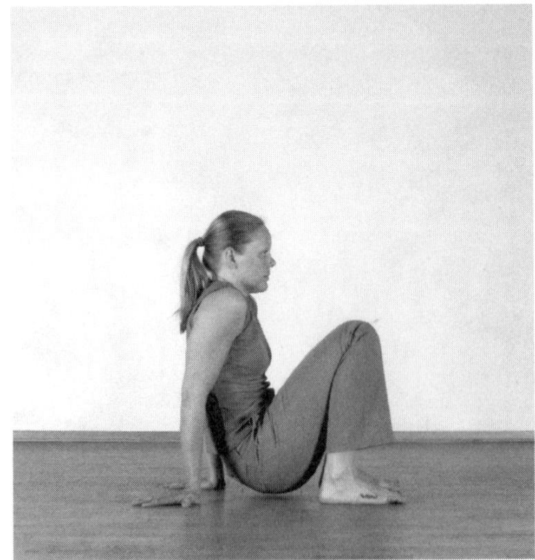

Breathing

Inhale in queda de quatro and exhale as you thrust up into the chapa kick. Or you can hold the movement at the top of the kick and remain static for 5 or 6 deep inhalations and exhalations while in the chapa position. In the latter exercise, just remember to exhale on the way up and inhale on the way down.

Pointers

Thrust your hips as high as you can and straighten your kicking leg.

Health and Fitness Benefits

Here the front of your body is given a strong stretch along its whole length. This stimulates your circulatory system and is a fantastic stretch for your legs, chest, shoulders, and abdomen. The mobility of your pelvis will be improved, and a full front-body stretch is beneficial for toning the nervous system.

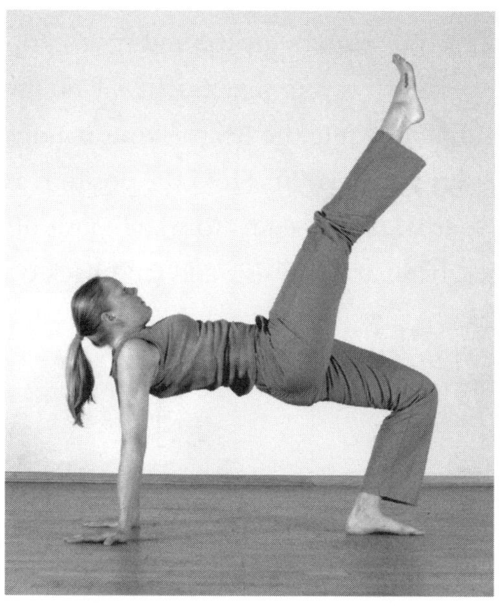

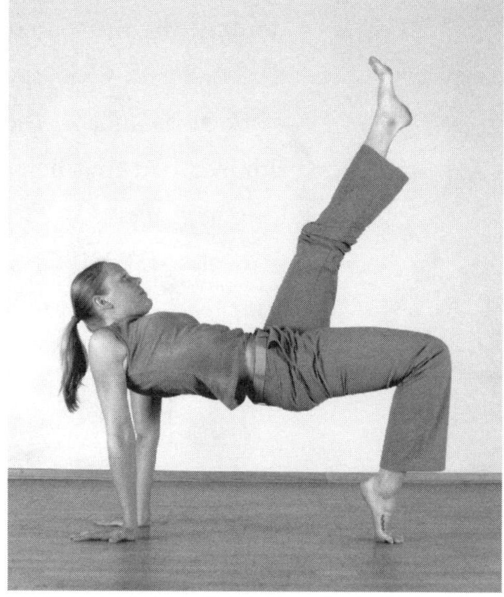

33. Plantanda Bananeira (handstand)

Strength. Balance.

Movement

Plantanda bananeira in capoeira means to plant a banana tree. It's a handstand. Do this movement against the wall for training, and as you build strength and balance, you can work away from the wall. Place your hands in front of the wall about 5 to 10 inches away from it, fingertips facing the wall and hands shoulder-width apart. Push up into a handstand with your heels resting against the wall, legs straight, body straight and in full alignment, head facing forward between your arms. Hold the position for 10 deep breaths.

Breathing

Breathe deeply through the nose.

Pointers

Stay centered and don't allow your legs to lean to one side while holding the movement. Keep your elbows locked and try to grip the floor with wide-open fingertips. It is your fingers that will do the work of balance in this handstand, while the heel of your hand is simply a pad that helps support your weight. Hold the position as long as it feels OK; when your strength begins to wane, push off from the wall with your feet, bend at the waist, and land back on your feet as lightly as you can.

Health and Fitness Benefits

Your spine is limbered up, arm and shoulder strength increase, and you also work your abdominal muscles. An excellent torso strength exercise, and as so many movements in capoeira are inverted, bananeira is useful for balance. The handstand is primary training for many gymnastic movements and is subsequently central to gymnastic and acrobatic training. Static inverted postures are also excellent for the circulation when combined with deep breathing.

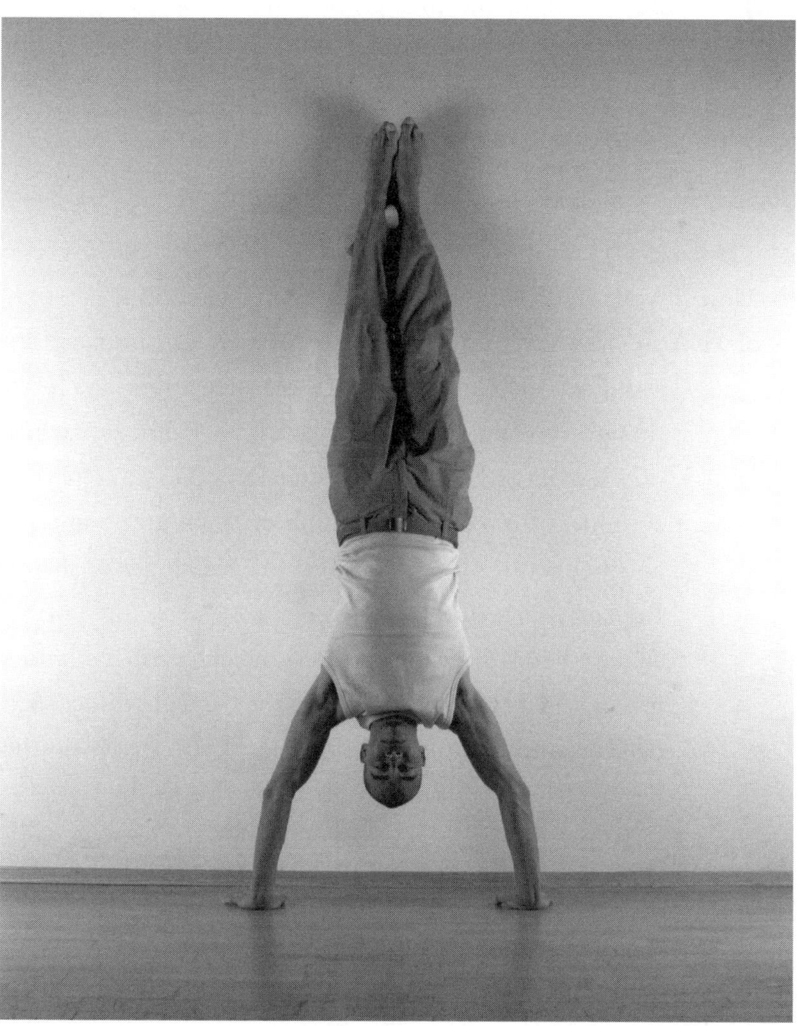

34. Bananeira Push-Up

Power. Strength. Balance. Agility.

Movement

Do a bananeira (No. 33) against the wall. Slowly lower yourself until the crown of your head touches the ground lightly. Immediately push up into the bananeira again, with your elbows locked. Keep your body straight and in alignment the whole time.

Breathing

Inhale on the way down; exhale on the way up.

Pointers

Always leave a repetition in reserve, and try not to do this exercise to failure. If you can do 3 reps, do 2 instead. If you can do 12, do only 10 or 11. You can always maximize your total reps by doing more sets. For example, do a set of 5 bananeira push-ups (even though you could probably manage 7). Come down and do a few cocorinha squats or stretches while you rest your shoulders for a couple of minutes, then go up and do another set of 5 repetitions of the bananeira push-up. Repeat this whole sequence for 10 sets and you've achieved 50 repetitions of the bananeira push-up (and a few hundred cocorinha squats in the bargain), rather than half the amount you might manage if you always do the reps to failure for each set.

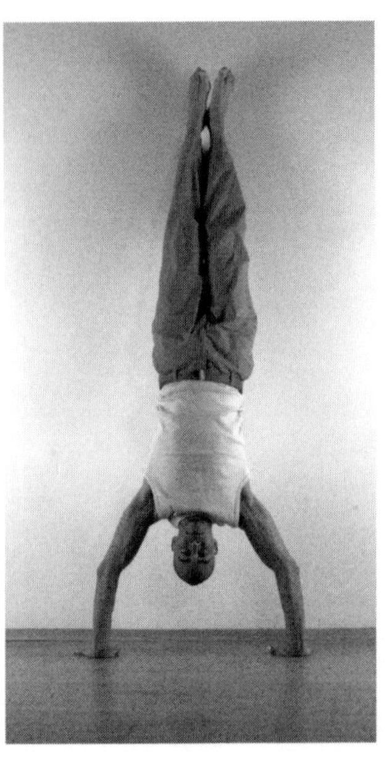

Note: As soon as your head touches the ground, push up; if you hang around down there resting weight on your head, it is much more difficult to push up.

Safety note: Do not dive-bomb the ground with the top of your head or you may injure your neck. Lower yourself slowly and steadily, concentrating on your breathing. If you can't do a single bananeira push-up, simply do a bananeira handstand and slowly lower yourself until the crown of your head makes contact with the floor. When this happens drop your feet to the floor gently and stand up. The act of lowering your body weight in a controlled way will increase your strength until you are ready for the full bananeira push-up.

Health and Fitness Benefits

This exercise is super-effective for building power in your torso. Your fingers, arms, chest, back, shoulders, and abdominal muscles are all worked, and if you practice the bananeira push-up faithfully you will notice improvements in your balance and in all cartwheel and inverted movements in capoeira. The benefits of this type of push-up can't be overstated; it's just an incredibly effective way of increasing your upper-body strength.

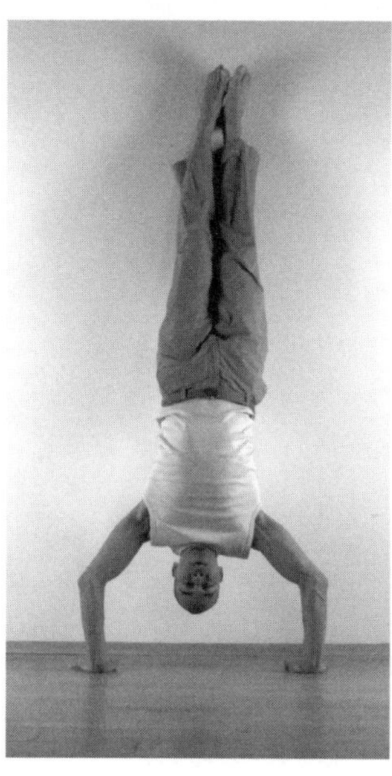
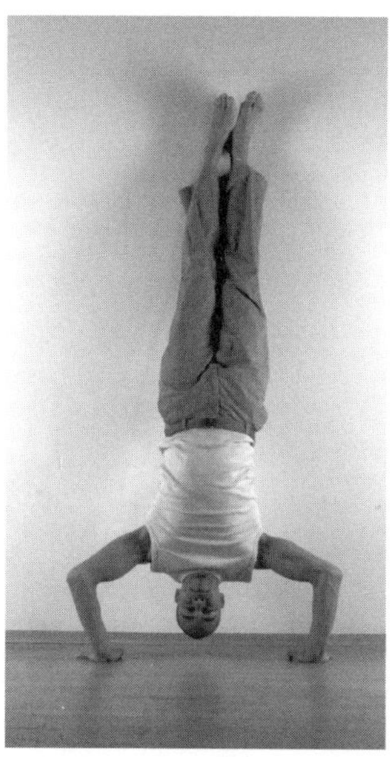
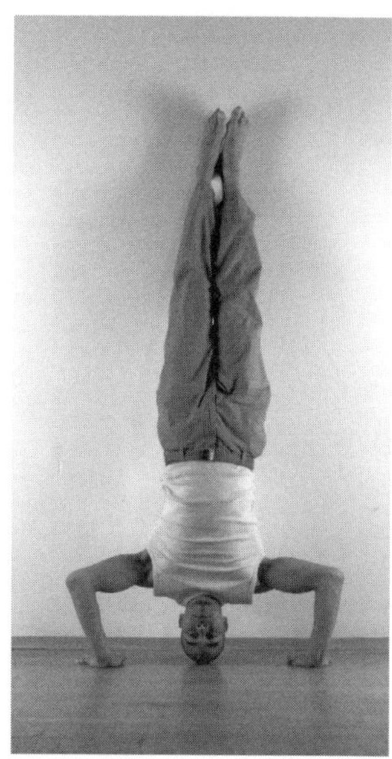

35. Bananeira Leg Stretch

Flexibility-stretch. Strength. Balance.

Movement

Do a bananeira and drop your legs to either side. Hold the position for 6 to 10 deep breaths.

Breathing

Regular deep nasal breathing.

Pointers

Hold your body stable and don't lean to one side. As you exhale, feel your legs opening wider as you relax the muscles. Try to hold the position for a couple of minutes if you can.

Health and Fitness Benefits

This will stretch the muscles of your inner thigh and groin, giving you greater flexibility for various capoeira kicks. The handstand will also increase strength in your upper body.

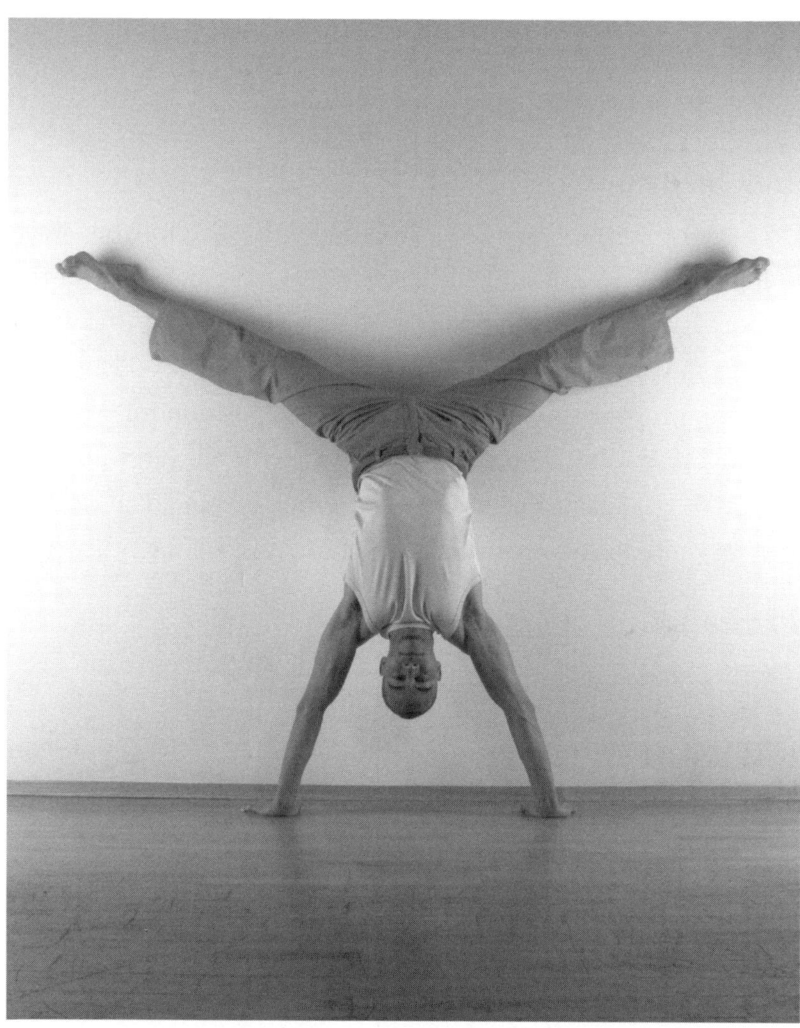

36. Queda de Rins

Strength. Balance.

Movement

Do the aú warm-up (No. 24). Drop down slowly until your waist or hip bone is resting on your inside elbow. The fingertips of the support hand on which you are resting will be facing backward, away from your body. Bring in both knees until your body weight is resting on your support elbow. Hold the position for a couple of deep breaths and then push back up into the aú warm-up position (No. 24) again. Flip over to the other side in an aú normal (No. 25) and do the same thing (queda de rins) on the other side.

Breathing

Breathe freely.

Pointers

Always warm up your wrists before this movement. Don't allow your elbow to slip up behind your back, but keep it slotted right into your waist so that it can support your weight. When you do the queda de rins, bring your knees together and rest securely, breathing deeply.

Health and Fitness Benefits

A good exercise for strengthening your wrists and for balance. The static movement will train your body for other types of aú queda de rins that are often used in the game of capoeira.

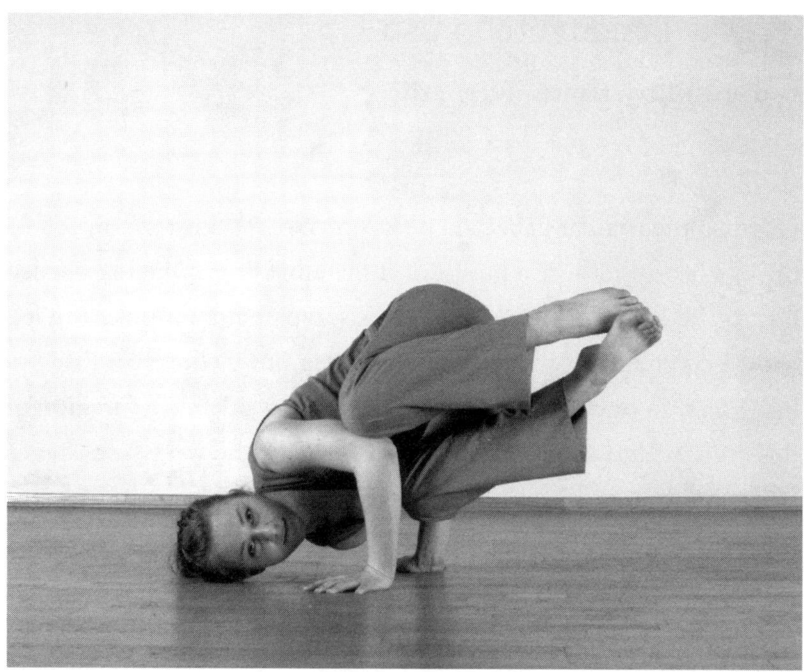

37. Leg Stretch Push-Ups

Flexibility-stretch. Strength.

Movement

Get into the regular cabeçada position (No. 9). Lower yourself to the bottom position of a push-up, at the same time swinging one leg out to the side along the ground. Rise up again and take the leg back. Lower again, swinging the other leg out to the side. Rise up, bringing it in once more. Repeat from side to side. As a variation of this exercise and to maximize the difficulty of the weight resistance (to increase strength and balance), each time you change legs, put the arm that's on the same side as the outside leg behind your back and do one-arm push-ups.

Breathing

Inhale on the way down and exhale on the way up.

Pointers

Touch your chest to the floor but don't lie on the floor. Swing your leg out as far as it will go to maximize your stretch. Keep your body aligned and stable as you move up and down in the push-up.

Health and Fitness Benefits

As with any push-up, this movement will work your chest, shoulders, back, and arms. The side swing will also stretch the inside of your legs.

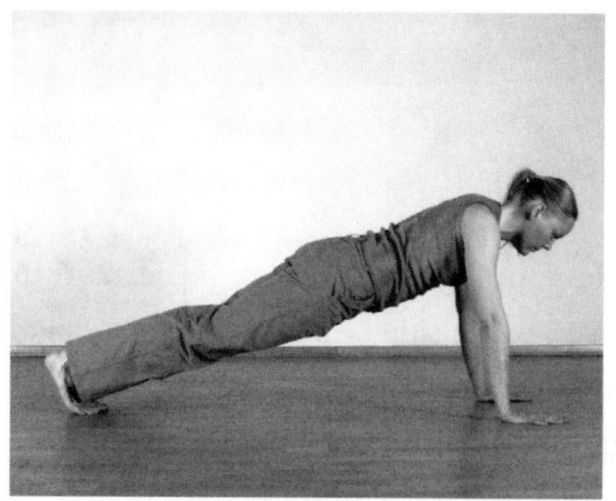
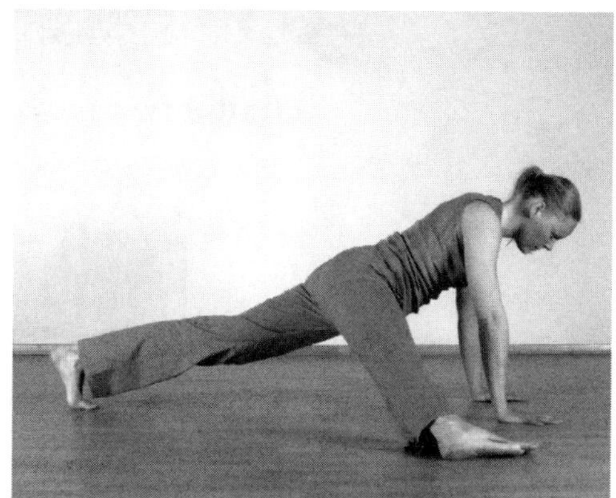
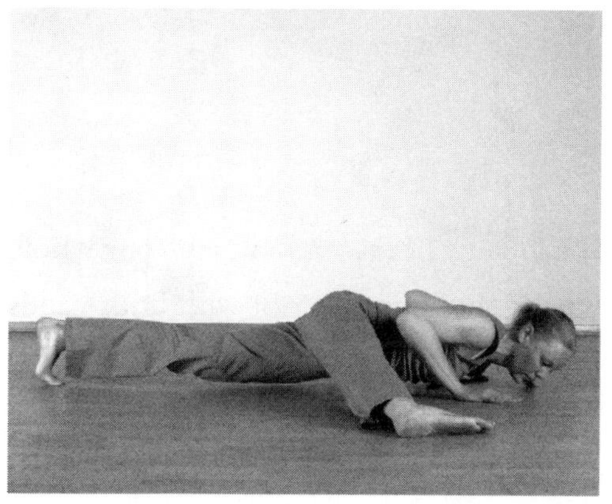
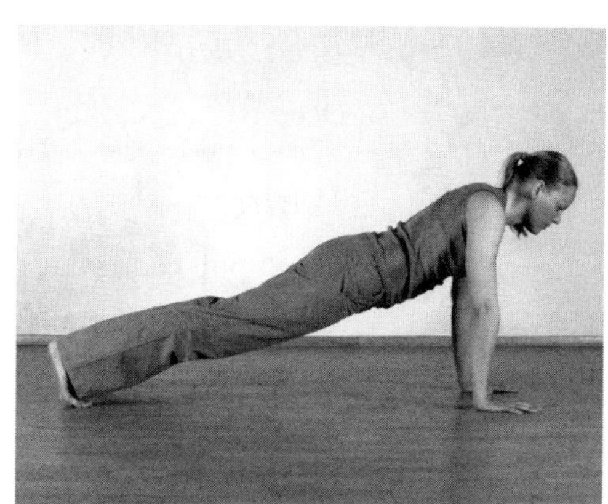
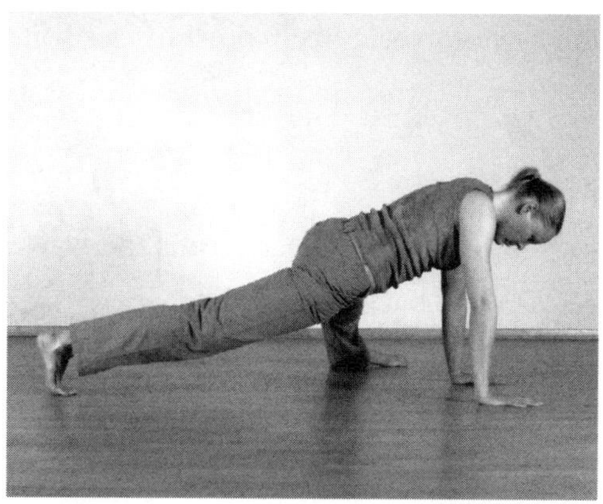
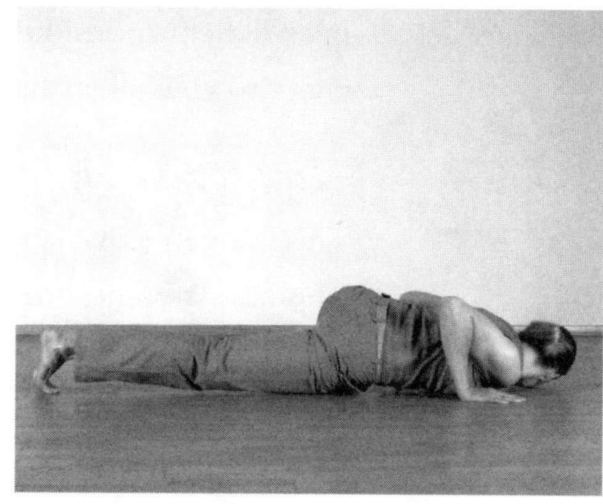

38. Side Split Twists

Flexibility-stretch.

Movement

Sit on the floor and spread your legs as widely as you can. Your toes can be either pointed out to the side or pointed at the ceiling. Bend to one side and grab your foot with both hands, keeping your chest pointing to the front. Take 6 deep breaths and then come up slowly and stretch to the other side, repeating the stretch.

Breathing

Deep nasal breathing.

Pointers

Try to pull back your toes, push your heels out, and lay your whole torso along the length of your leg, holding the foot with both hands to increase the side stretch. Your ear can be lying on your shin by the end of the completed movement. Ease into the stretch and don't attempt to force yourself into a position by hunching over forward or forcing yourself beyond what is comfortable. Breathing will help enormously, and as you exhale, feel your muscles softening so you fall farther into the fully stretched-out side split twist.

Health and Fitness Benefits

This is an effective lateral stretch for your spine. It trims the waist. This also stretches the muscles at the back of your legs, increasing your range of movement for kicks like queixada, armada, martelo, chapa, and so on.

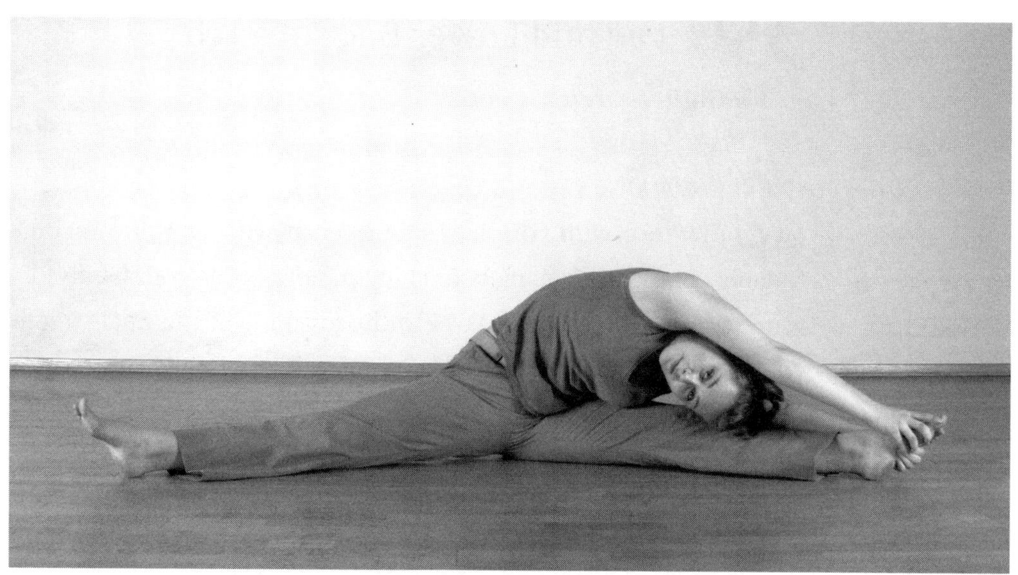

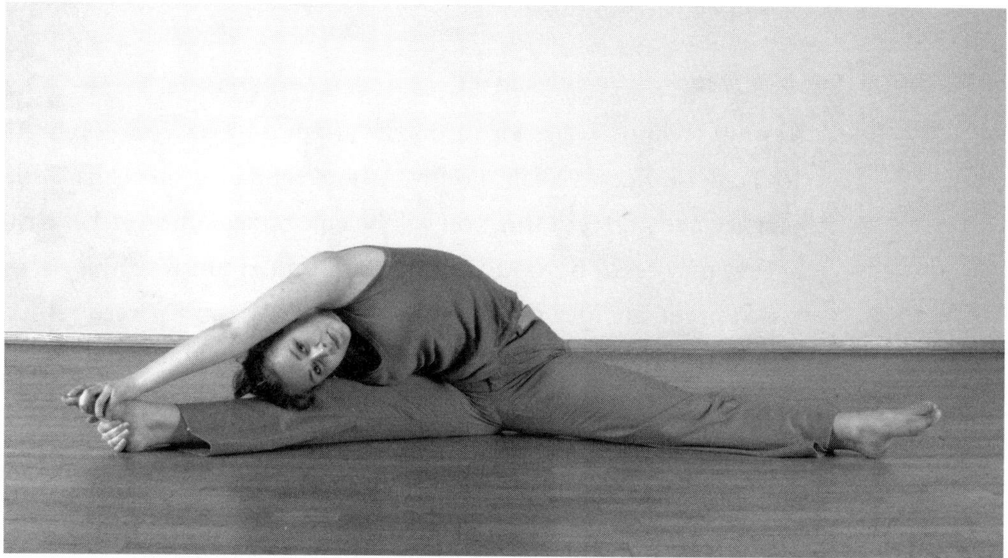

39. Leg and Lower Back Stretch

Flexibility-stretch.

Movement

Sit on the floor with your legs split open as wide as you can comfortably get them. Keeping your chin up, slowly walk your hands forward, trying to take your navel to the ground. In the final stretch your whole trunk, from navel to chin, will be resting forward on the ground, with your arms outstretched in front of you.

Breathing

Deep nasal breathing. Allow gravity to help you as you imagine your lower back and inner thighs softening, sinking farther forward as you exhale fully.

Pointers

Try not to hunch over forward in an attempt to get your forehead to the floor. Keep a totally positive attitude and remember that with practice and correct form, you will be able to achieve stretches that at first may seem beyond your reach. Don't strain with this exercise. Forget the idea of "no pain, no gain." Work forward rather than downward and never force the stretch until you feel uncomfortable pain.

Health and Fitness Benefits

A great full-body stretch for your lower back, upper back, legs, and chest. As with the side split twists (No. 38), this will increase flexibility for a wide range of capoeira techniques.

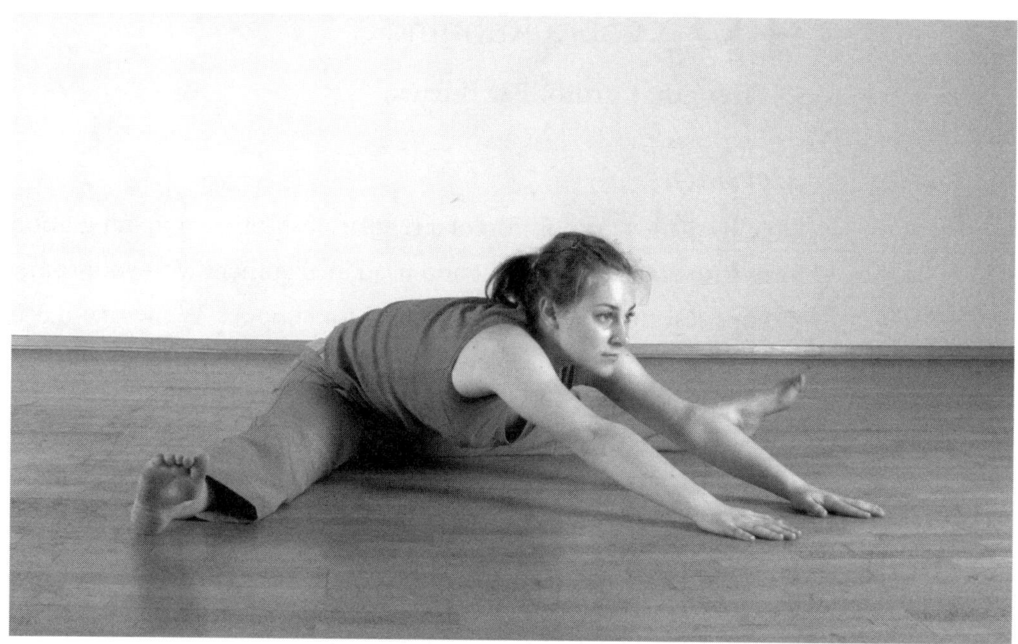

40. Cobra Running

Strength. Cardio. Fat Burner.

Movement

Go into the lowest position of a regular push-up, maintaining good form with your back straight and head in alignment with your spine. Do not rest the chest on the ground for support. While maintaining this position, run in place on your toes for 10 or 20 steps, then stop and push up.

Breathing

Breathe freely.

Pointers

Run rapidly, keep your elbows in, and don't bang your chin on the ground. This can be effectively combined with a no cheat bridge (No. 20). (See the Workout Menu.)

Health and Fitness Benefits

This is good cardiovascular training and is strengthening for your chest, arms, legs, lungs, and heart. It builds speed and springiness in the legs and arms.

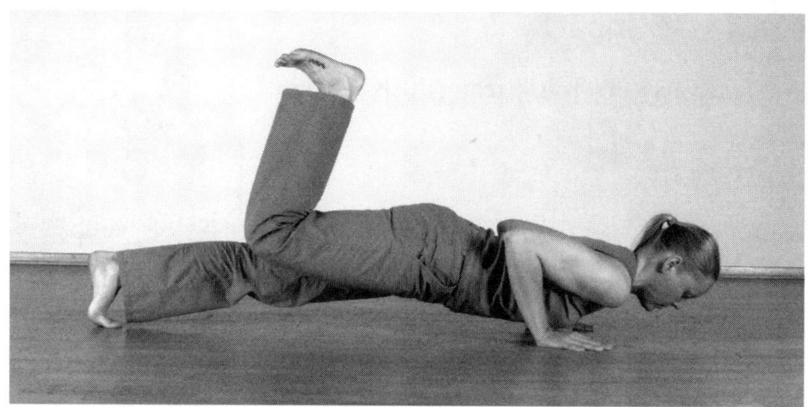

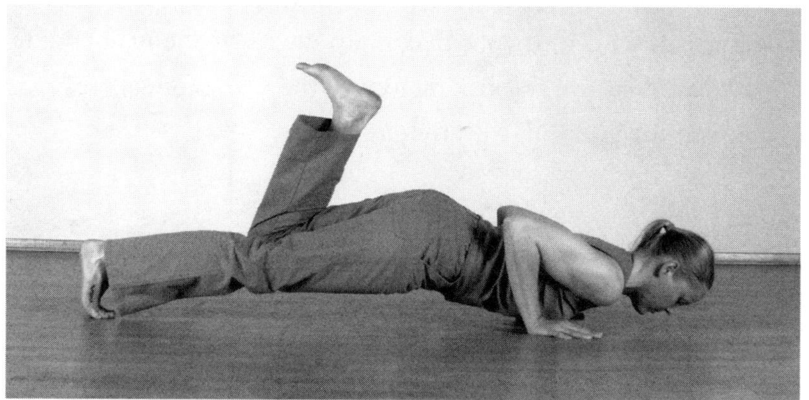

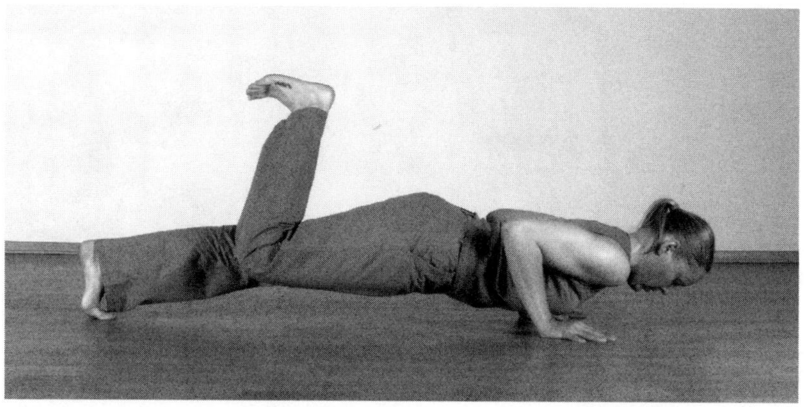

41. Bênção

Flexibility-stretch. Strength. Balance.

Movement

This is a front kick delivered from a ginga. The kicking leg is back in a ginga, then the back leg is raised, with the knee high and directly in front of the body. The arms come out to the sides, with the hands relaxed and open. To execute the kick, thrust forward with the hips and straighten out the kicking leg simultaneously, drawing the toes back so that the kicking surface is the sole of the foot. Once you have thrust forward to your maximum degree while maintaining good balance, return the kicking foot to the rear, original position, ginga, and then bênção with the other leg.

Breathing

Exhale as you kick for maximum power and balance; otherwise breathe freely during the ginga stage.

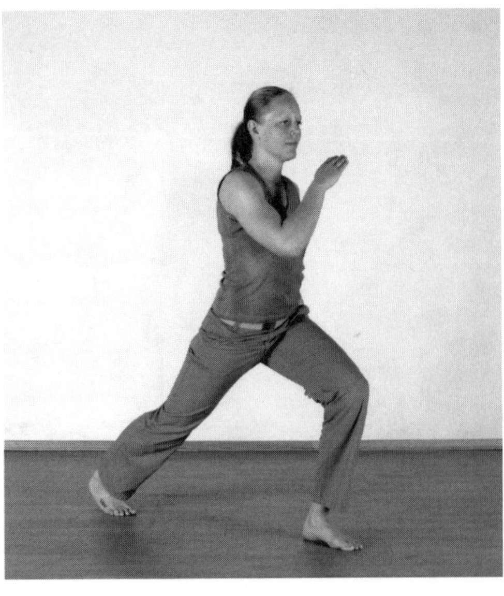

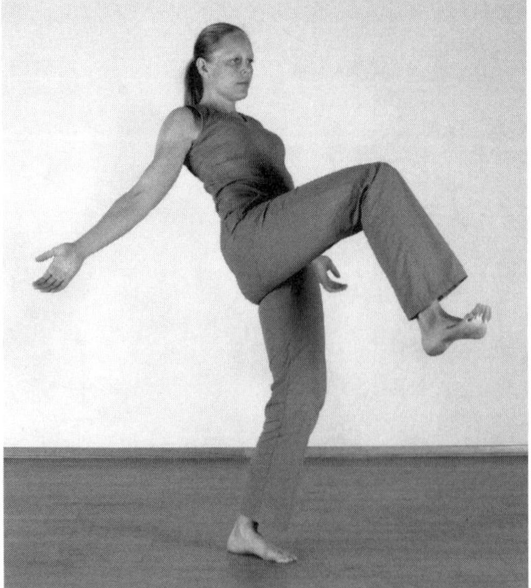

Pointers

Drive your hips upward and forward after you have raised the knee. Keep your supporting foot flat on the ground. You can do this kick fast and repeat it for multiple reps, or do it in slow motion to increase your balance and work on controlling your raised kicking leg without hopping about, but remaining rooted and stable on your support leg.

Health and Fitness Benefits

This will increase your balance and gives a good workout to the hips and lower back. It also exercises the abdominal muscles, which are used to stabilize the body in the kicking position. The abs are the hinge between the upper and lower body, and many fast-paced but controlled reps or a slow and concentrated static control while in the kicking position will work the abs.

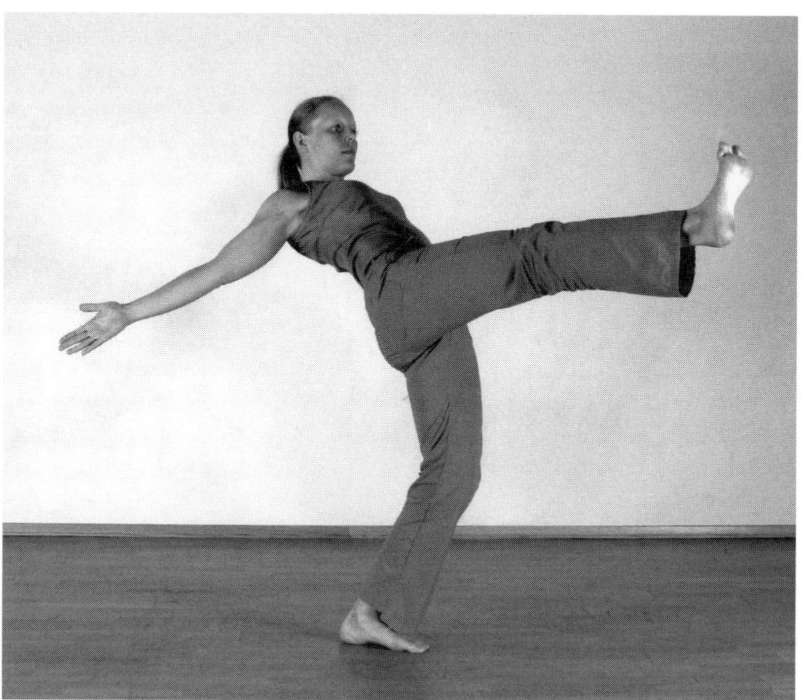

Chapter 4

Questions and Answers

How often can I train?

You can do capoeira conditioning training every day. There's nothing in the whole schedule that can't be done back-to-back on an every day of the week basis if that's what you feel like.

What and how should I eat?

As with any fitness program you'll have much more energy if you eat healthy food in the right combination. Some good ideas are to:

- Wait about four hours between meals.
- Wait around 60 to 90 minutes after eating before you do capoeira conditioning exercises.
- Eat plenty of fruit and vegetables. About five portions a day are recommended. When it's convenient, try not to mix concentrated starch and protein at the same meal, as that will make you sluggish. Meat and potatoes taste great together, but you're going to know about it when you try bridge walking after lunch. Avoid processed food and sugary drinks like soda. Try not to eat too much sugar, especially before training.
- Drink plenty of water, preferably 8 glasses (64 oz.) a day.

Drink before you eat or at least half an hour after you've eaten. If you feel wilting and fatigued, it might be that you're not drinking enough water, so put water at the top of your priority list. It is a good habit to drink at least one pint of water upon waking in the morning.

Incidentally, on the subject of food for physical performance, there is ample evidence that reducing or even eliminating meat from the diet altogether can have overall benefits for health and recovery after exercise. Fish is easier to digest and lower in saturated fat than red meat. Oily fish like salmon or trout give a good supply of long-chain omega-3 fatty acids, which are vital for maintaining a healthy central nervous system. Vegetarian sources of omega-3 can be gained from flax seeds and walnuts. The list of world class athletes who are vegetarian or vegan is long and distinguished. Both endurance and power athletes are represented.

At his athletic peak, multi-gold-medal-winning Olympic sprinter and long jumper Carl Lewis was a vegan (meaning he ate no meat, fish, cheese, milk, butter, or eggs). He remains a vegan today. Hawaiian Dr. Ruth Heidrich, at 70 years of age, is still a superfit competitor and age-group record holder at the finish line of the grueling Ironman Triathlon. She is also a vegan. Triathlon legend and six-time Ironman Triathlon winner Dave Scott is a vegan. Tennis champion Martina Navratilova was and is a vegan. World Trampoline champion and U.S. national champion gymnast Dan Millman is a vegan. Power athletes and world class bodybuilders Bill Pearl and Albert Beckles are both vegetarian. Incredibly, Beckles, who was born in 1930, continued to win top-class professional championships into the 1990s on a vegetarian diet. If that isn't longevity in sport, then nothing is. In the fighting arts, Ridgely Abele, winner of eight U.S. national championships in karate, is a vegetarian.

Although it is perfectly possible to eat a healthy diet containing a ***moderate*** quantity of meat, it is also a fact that many well-controlled scientific studies done on vegetarian groups such as Seventh Day Adventists have consistently demonstrated a reduced risk of obesity, heart disease, hypertension (high blood pressure), stroke, arthritis, and certain types of cancer among vegans and vegetarians. If you do decide to go vegetarian, make sure you eat a balanced, varied diet with plenty of green, leafy vegetables, legumes, nuts, grains, and protein products like soy milk or tofu. As long as you don't overdo it on the dairy products, a vegetarian diet ensures an immediate drop in dietary saturated fat, which is a gift to your heart.

Raw fruit and vegetable juice is a healthy option too and you can always dump a couple of spoonfuls of soy powder, tofu, tahini, or nut butter in there if you want to fortify them with protein. To retain all the fiber in juice smoothies, peel and core fruits like apples and pears and use the whole fruit in the blender, added to frozen bananas, frozen blueberries, strawberries, avocados, vegetable juices, barley malt, or soy milk. The list of goodies is endless and will give you an incredible energy boost if drunk a half hour or so before capoeira conditioning training. If you train hard regularly you might also try a daily multi vitamin and mineral tablet and an iron and B-vitamin supplement. This is also true for nonvegetarians who are involved in regular active physical training. The bottom line is that the combination of regular exercise and a healthy diet is the best health insurance you can get.

Will I lose weight?

If you do capoeira conditioning regularly and eat sensibly then you'll burn a lot more calories than if you do nothing, let's put it that way. Check out the fat burners in the Training Effects Chart for accelerated calorie consumption.

Will capoeira conditioning improve my sex life?

Yes. (Only joking. That's up to you.)

How long should I train every day?

How fit do you want to be? Fifteen minutes a day is a minimum and will build and maintain a reasonable level of conditioning. If that is what you have time for, then we would suggest that 15 minutes of capoeira conditioning is a more holistic and well-balanced exercise investment than 15 minutes running or weight training.

If you can find time to do longer sessions, say a 30- or 45-minute session once or twice a week, that will also be great for your fitness gains. Remember, six days of nothing will not be replaced effectively by one and a half hours' training on the seventh day. Regularity is the best, and 15 minutes of varied capoeira conditioning per day is enough to keep the machine ticking.

Can I get as strong doing capoeira conditioning as I can doing weight training or bodybuilding?

Strength is relative to what you want. If you want to bench-press 400 pounds, then you'll have to do something additional to capoeira conditioning. If you want to handle your body weight well in different positions, to be supple, agile, strong but also fluid, well-balanced, and aerobically fit, then you can certainly get as much from capoeira conditioning as from bodybuilding.

I am 45 years old and I haven't trained since I was in my 20s. Can I do this?

Absolutely. You have everything to gain and nothing to lose by beginning immediately. Remember to consult your physician before you start this exercise program and then begin slowly with the 7½-minute sessions done at a steady "aerobic" pace. You will be amazed at your progress and how much better you feel after a few weeks of these exercises. Mestre Pastinha, one of the legends of capoeira, was still incredibly lithe, slim, and fit as a fiddle when he was in his 70s.

Some of the exercises look impossible. Is capoeira really for me?

Stick to the exercises you feel comfortable with. As your body loosens up, your strength will increase (as well as your confidence) and you will find you will want to sneak in some of the exercises that look unusual (and there aren't that many of those). One by one you will see how the "impossible" becomes possible.

Can children do this stuff?

Yes, children love standing on their hands (bananeira), cartwheels (aú), and bridging. Just watch out for the furniture and your knick-knacks. Stiffness and postural problems set in early in these days of TV and computer games, so working their bodies through a range of natural movements is one of the finest things children can do to grow up healthy, strong, and well.

What about music?

Do these exercises to music, definitely. Purists may want to stick Mestre João Grande or Mestre Sombra into their iPod, but these exercises are fun to do to any music, and as capoeira is a fight-dance-game that is done to music, go for it.

About the Author

Gerard Taylor is one of the first generation of non-Brazilian students who have benefited from capoeira's establishment in Europe. After having been totally sold on the fitness boom of the late 1970s, he first heard of capoeira in the mid 1980s and began training in Britain's first capoeira school, The London School of Capoeira, in 1989. He trained three to four times a week with Master Sylvia Bazzarelli and Contra Master Marcos Dos Santos for the next seven years, before moving to Oslo, Norway, where he co-founded the Oslo Capoeira Klubb with Agnes Folkestad, another of the LSC's students. Since 1996 Taylor has taught capoeira classes and workshops to thousands of people of all ages and many nationalities. From this experience he has developed a teaching and fitness method that works effectively for adults and children alike.

Capoeira Conditioning is Taylor's second book about this popular martial art. His first book, *Capoeira: The Jogo de Angola from Luanda to Cyberspace,* Volume One (North Atlantic Books, 2005), is a comprehensive history of capoeira, tracing its foundations in central African martial traditions to its development into a fighting art in colonial Brazil. Volume Two, to be published by Blue Snake Books in 2006, will detail capoeira's transition into Brazil's national sport and its explosive growth worldwide.

Since the late 1970s Gerard has worked in various fields of journalism and copywriting, including for the Foundation for African

Arts, and as Northern Ireland editor for the *Black Voice* newspaper. More recently he has written text for theatre companies in London and for Apple Records on the Beatles1 official website. He is also finalizing work on a vegetarian and vegan cookbook, and has recently finished an encyclopedic history of Los Angeles and San Francisco punk rock music.

Anders Kjaergaard is a professional photographer living and working in London, England. In addition to shooting all the photographs in *Capoeira Conditioning,* he and Sue Parkhill illustrated Taylor's previous book, *Capoeira: The Jogo de Angola from Luanda to Cyberspace,* Volume One.

Kjaergaard and Parkhill are both graduates of the Royal College of Art, where they studied photography on the MA program. They both continue to show their own work internationally as well as collaborating on projects such as this one.